AN ATLAS OF
MEDICAL
MICROBIOLOGY
COMMON HUMAN
PATHOGENS

AN ATLAS OF MEDICAL MICROBIOLOGY

COMMON HUMAN PATHOGENS

Bryan C. Stratford

ED, MD(Melb), FRACP, FRCPA, MRCPath(Eng)
Director of Microbiology, St. Vincent's Hospital,
Melbourne, Australia
Senior Associate, Department of
Microbiology, University of Melbourne
Formerly Part-time Teaching Staff, Department of
Microbiology, Monash University, Melbourne
Consultant Microbiologist, Hospitals and
Charities Commission of Victoria

Blackwell Scientific Publications

OXFORD LONDON EDINBURGH MELBOURNE

Distributed in the United States of
America by J.B. Lippincott Company,
Philadelphia,
and in Canada by
J.B. Lippincott Company of Canada
Ltd, Toronto

Origination by
Typesetting Services Ltd
Glasgow
Printed and bound in
Great Britain by
Morrison & Gibb Ltd
Edinburgh

First published 1977

Stratford, Bryan C
An atlas of medical microbiology:
common human pathogens
Bibl.—Index.
ISBN 0–632–00398–7
1. Title
616.01   QR46
Medical microbiology

FOREWORD BY

William Brumfitt

MD, PhD, FRCP, FRCPath,
Professor of Medical Microbiology
in the University of London
Chairman of the Division of
Pathology and Head of the
Department of Microbiology
The Royal Free Hospital, London

Contents

SECTION III. SYSTEMATIC
BACTERIOLOGY

SECTION IV. MYCOLOGY

Foreword

Medical microbiology is both an art and a science and, as is well known, the latter is easier to teach than the former. To hold the interest and fire the imagination of students of this subject, first-class demonstration material is always essential.

Unfortunately with increasing pressure on laboratory staff, such preparations are tending to become the exception rather than the rule. Another limiting factor is the lack of fresh material, particularly those exotic diseases which are being seen more often world wide—especially with shifting populations and rapid forms of transport.

Anybody concerned with demonstrating medical microbiology is well aware that even a superb preparation may rapidly deteriorate, to the chagrin of pupil and teacher alike. Thus a permanent record of such a wide selection of material, covering all aspects of the subject, will be of inestimable value. Those benefiting will not only be persons directly concerned with microbiology, but also practitioners in numerous branches of medicine upon which the subject impinges.

However, this endeavour would largely fail if it were not compiled by a worker with extensive knowledge of both the clinical and laboratory aspects of medical microbiology. Dr Bryan Stratford has shown that he is admirably suited to carry out this major undertaking. Other excellent illustrated texts have appeared, but none is so comprehensive as this book.

One obvious advantage of such a work is that, unlike textbooks, which rapidly become out-dated, this volume will be as valuable in ten years time as it is today. We must be grateful to Dr Stratford and his indefatigable colleagues for giving this fascinating record of their experience acquired over many years and assembled with great care.

William Brumfitt

Preface

The aim of this book is to present in pictorial fashion a companion volume to any of the recognized textbooks of microbiology where photographs are often lacking. The written word is kept to a minimum. The book does not pretend in any way to be a textbook of microbiology.

An important section is that concerning 'Collection of Specimens' which must involve nurses, junior doctors and medical students. The remainder of the volume is devoted to the visual representation of various microorganisms, fungi, viruses, and common parasites. All of those shown in the text can present to a routine hospital laboratory service.

The book is directed mainly to medical students, science students majoring in micro-

biology, and, of course, medical technologists, whether trained or in training. But it is hoped that hospital, university and nursing school libraries will find it of value.

With few exceptions, references are not included in the text. Where they do appear they are key references and the reader is advised to consult them.

It should be stressed that, as the name of the book suggests, it deals with common human pathogens, thus rare diseases are not included.

I wish to thank a number of people without whose help this volume could not have been completed. First Mrs Shirley Dixson, BSc, whose help in the preparation of the bacteriological specimens has been invaluable. Miss

Cathy Lee, also from my laboratory, prepared most of the specimens in the mycology section. Another helper in mycology was Miss G. Brown from the Children's Hospital in Adelaide. Both Dr G. Tannock from the Commonwealth Serum Laboratories and Dr Ian Gust from Fairfield Hospital contributed to the virology sections, and Dr G. Buist from the same hospital helped with syphilis serology. Dr Gust also kindly supplied Figs. VII.3 to 7. Mr D. R. McDonald photographed Figs. IV.7 to 10, 15, 16, 20, 21 and 23. Major Bryce Redington, PhD, USA, MC, gave expert help in the Parasitology Section. Mr. Mario Cotela, Clinical Photographer at St Vincent's Hospital, Melbourne, deserves great credit for his efforts. Equally, I am grateful for the help I have received at the Armed Forces Institute of Pathology, Washington, DC, both in the Parasitology Section with its photographs, but also for the amenities which have allowed me to complete the book. Finally, the late Professor G. C. de Gruchy, Professor S. Faine and Professor D. Penington kindly read all or part of the manuscript and gave enormous help. Lastly, my thanks go to my wife, Dr Bernice Stratford, and Dr David Leslie, who not only corrected my grammar, but also painstakingly read the page proofs.

Melbourne, July 1976

Acknowledgments

The author wishes to express his gratitude to Roussel Pharmaceuticals (Aust) Ltd for a substantial donation towards the cost of this book.

Other companies whom I wish to thank are:
Beecham Research Laboratories (Aust) Ltd,
Lederle (Cyanamid Aust) Ltd,
Ensign Laboratories (Aust) Ltd,
Denver Laboratories (Aust) Pty Ltd,
Glaxo Holdings (Eng) Ltd,
Eli Lilly Pty Ltd,
Ultra-Violet Supplies Ltd,
Oliphant Industries Ltd,
ICI (Aust) Ltd,
A. E. Stansen & Co Ltd.

Without the financial assistance of these various companies it would have been impossible to keep the price of this book within reasonable bounds so that a student could afford it.

SECTION I
GENERAL
INTRODUCTION

Introduction

This book lays emphasis on the practical and in particular the visual aspects of the laboratory diagnosis of microbial diseases. So far as is possible details of laboratory procedures are omitted. These can be obtained from recommended textbooks. However, many of these lack the illustrations to demonstrate their written facts. The section on Collection of Specimens is important, because without correct specimen collection the laboratory cannot provide a meaningful result.

This book is an attempt to supplement in pictorial fashion most of the common specimens seen in medical microbiology. Some repetition is unavoidable, but is kept to a minimum. Stress is placed on the collection and in some instances, the treatment of specimens.

The section on Systematic Bacteriology is necessarily the largest. In this and all other sections no photograph has been 'touched up'. What is seen in the illustration is what one actually sees. Magnifications are given with the photomicrographs, so the correct magnification must be used to compare similar preparations.

The major blastomycoses are rare in this country so few are mentioned.

No one could present such an atlas and satisfy everybody. Media considered important by some workers are only mentioned or not shown at all. Those illustrated are in common use and have been shown satisfactory for most purposes of identification.

Recommendations throughout are for the use of disposable items of equipment, e.g. gloves, masks, tongue depressors, syringes and many other articles. These are preferable to items designed to last, as the use of 'disposables' cuts out the necessity for cleaning and resterilization which are expensive both of time and effort.

Illustrations are numbered according to their sections, e.g. II.3 is the third photograph in Section II, i.e. in the Section referring to Collection of Specimens.

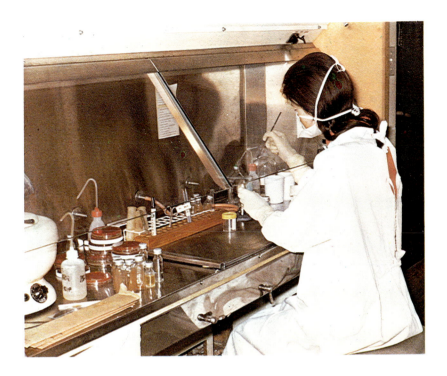

Fig. I.1. Normal T.B. or safety cabinet. Note that all the items required for work are enclosed in the cabinet and further that only the workers' *arms* protrude below the safety glass partition.

Chapter 1
Safety in the Laboratory

Many workers in routine laboratories do not realize that they work with specimens potentially hazardous to their own health. In general, it is only with tuberculosis material that special care is taken. Rightly so, but tuberculosis is becoming a rare disease!

The majority of laboratories use a safety cabinet for T.B. work. Such cabinets are normally glass-faced to prevent accidental spillage above the level of the worker's chest (Fig. I.1). In addition, the technician wears gloves, gown and a mask to minimize laboratory infection.

Although such cabinets and precautions are neither available nor necessary for processing most specimens in the routine laboratory, it should not be forgotten that a drop of infected urine is equivalent to a drop of pus. Specimens thought to contain highly pathogenic or communicable organisms, e.g. anthrax, should be handled in a safety cabinet with full precautions.

In parts of the laboratory dealing with blood products the risk of contracting hepatitis is rare but nevertheless real. It warrants special care and the use of gloves together with liquid formalin disinfection.

Mouth pipettes should not be used because infected material may be inadvertently sucked up. Rubber safety bulbs should be employed. Aerosols present the most danger in any laboratory and the 'coronet' effect of a spilled drop is shown in Fig. I.2, and the 'string of pearls' aerosol associated with blowing out a pipette is

Fig. I.2. 'Coronet effect' of a drop spilled on glass. This photograph shows the classical coronet type of aerosol dispersal consequent on a spilled drop of fluid. Many more microscopic particles are shed at the same time.

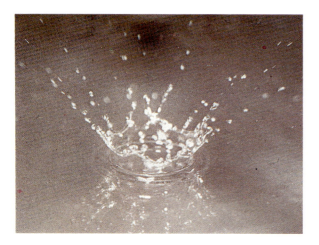

Fig. I.3. 'String of pearls' aerosol from a pipette being blown out. The analogy is sometimes hard to see, perhaps a 'diamond necklette' would be better. Again, note that the macroscopic droplets are but a fraction of the total aerosol expelled.

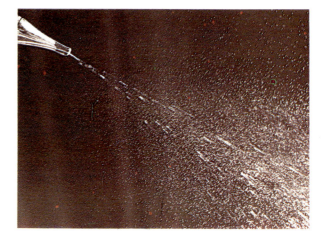

shown in Fig. I.3.

Hand to mouth transfer of bacteria readily occurs but is easily controlled. First, the worker can wear disposable gloves and a mask. Second, and less annoying, the use of an antibacterial hand lotion (see p. 6) to kill both transient and resident skin bacteria obviates this risk (Figs. I.4, I.5 and I.6).

Pressure or squeeze packs of formalin should be available for the disinfection of serology benches as a frequent routine. Another useful antibacterial pressure pack* contains 95 per cent alcohol and 1 per cent chlorhexidine (Hibitane®)

which can be used for 'flash' disinfection of solid surfaces (Figs. I.7 and I.8).

In the microbiology laboratory and its work areas, e.g. wash-up rooms, staff should wear long-sleeved, heavy duty twill gowns (NOT coats) as a protection over their clothes against spillage and aerosols (Fig. I.9).

Common sense and a knowledge of how materials may be hazardous is important. Corridors should be equipped with safety showers, asbestos blankets, sand buckets and appropriate fire extinguishers. Fire drill should be regularly rehearsed and there should be nominated fire wardens.

Smoking and eating in the laboratory must be absolutely forbidden.

---

*An antibacterial pressure pack, containing chlorhexidine in ethyl alcohol is obtainable from Ensign Laboratories, Wellington Road, Mulgrave, Victoria, 3170. Australia.

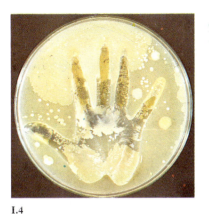

I.4

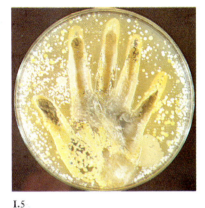

I.5

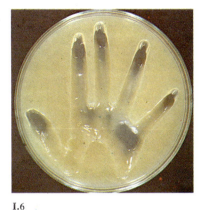

I.6

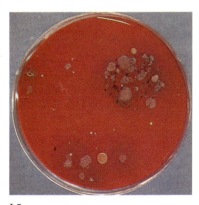

I.7

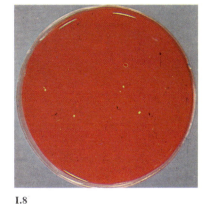

I.8

Fig. I.4. Impression plate of an unwashed hand. Obviously many organisms are present on the unwashed hand; most belong to the 'transient' or 'superficial' flora, but may still be pathogenic.

Fig. I.5. Impression plate of a hand following 5 min surgical scrub-up. In this picture the removal, by scrubbing, of the flora present in Fig. I.4 is well shown. This person is a hand carrier of *Staphylococcus aureus* in her 'deep' or 'resident' flora, and this organism now predominates. Thus, the surgical scrub does not eliminate pathogens but in susceptible people (10–20 per cent of normal) brings the pathogen to the surface!

Fig. I.6. Impression plate after use of the glove lotion—time 3 hours. This picture is of the same hand as in Fig. I.5 after use of the 'glove' lotion. The same effect is not seen if only the 'ward' lotion and no gloves are used.

Fig. I.7. Contact samples (3) cultured from a laboratory bench. The presence of many bacteria, only some of which are pathogenic, others being *Bacillus spp.* from dust, is well shown in this photograph.

Fig. I.8. Contact samples (3) cultured from a laboratory bench when dry after spraying with alcoholic chlorhexidine. Three velvet covered samples are used to show the 'flash'

disinfection due to the 75 per cent ethyl alcohol; the 1 per cent chlorhexidine gives a small measure of lasting effect.

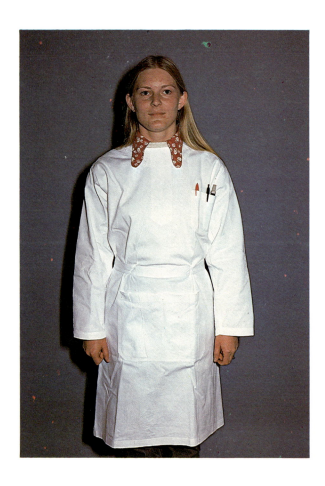

Fig. I.9. Protective gown for laboratory workers. The gown shown protects from obvious or accidental microscopic or macroscopic spillage. Being heavy duty twill cotton it is neither easily permeable nor readily flammable. Coats leave areas on the front of the worker unprotected.

Recommended Formulations of Hand Lotions

WARD LOTION

Chlorhexidine diacetate	1 %
Cetyl alcohol	0.7 %
Isopropyl alcohol	45 %
Isopropyl palmitate	1.4 %
Polyethylene oxide ('Polyox resin' WSR 205)	0.07 %
Ethyl alcohol (abs)	30 %
Distilled water to	100 %

LOTION FOR GLOVE USE

Chlorhexidine diacetate	1 %
Cetyl alcohol	1 %
Polyethylene oxide ('Polyox resin' WSR 205)	0.1 %
Isopropyl palmitate	2 %
Ethyl alcohol (abs)	15 %
Cetamacregol BCP	3 %
Polyethylene monolaurate	4 %
Terpineol	0.5 %
Isopropyl alcohol	40 %
Distilled water to	100 %

SECTION II
THE COLLECTION
OF SPECIMENS

Introduction

The proper collection of specimens and time of
their collection, the speed with which they are
transferred to the laboratory and their subsequent
handling all make for a correct microbiological
diagnosis. As a principle it can be stated that
saliva is no substitute for sputum, nor if urine
is left at room temperature for two hours or
longer can the colony count be considered
significant, as this time is enough to incubate and
give an artificially high colony count. Immediate
processing or refrigeration of urine specimens
obviates this risk and can show the organisms
to be mere contaminants. CSF specimens require urgent transport to the laboratory. If a cell
count is to be useful, it must be performed
within half an hour of collection. Swabs to

identify the gonococcus and the meningococcus have the same time restriction.

Swabs for clinical use are best dipped in homologous human serum* before sterilization as most organisms remain viable on them for 12–24 hours. In contrast, fastidious organisms quickly die on undipped cotton wool swabs. If there is any delay in processing, swabs should *not* be refrigerated.

If the specimen cannot be examined immediately for *Neisseria gonorrhoeae* infections, a charcoal swab and Stuart's medium retains viability of organisms for 48–72 hours. This set can be used for the transport of any micro-organism, see Chapter 16.

Current opinion is that not more than ten minutes should elapse between collection and processing of specimens for anaerobic culture.

The chapters which follow detail an acceptable method of collection and transport of specimens.

* Rubbo, S. D. & Benjamin, M. (1951) Some observations on survival of pathogenic bacteria on cotton-wool swabs. Development of a new type of swab. *Br. med. J.*, **1**, 983.

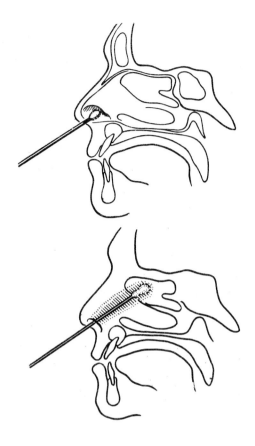

Fig. II.1. Procedure for taking a nasal swab. By this method *both* the anterior nares and the deeper recesses of the nose are sampled at the same time. Normally, one swab is used to sample both nostrils.

Chapter 2
Nasal Swabs

Technically, taking a nasal swab is not difficult, but it is often performed incorrectly. A common error is to swab only the external nares—mainly out of consideration for the patient's comfort.

It is more reasonable to expect organisms to be present in the deeper, moist, warmer recesses of the nose. It was shown at least 13 years ago in patients that a deep swab under the middle turbinate recovered 11 per cent more *Staphylococcus aureus* than did an anterior swab alone. Therefore, a combined anterior and deep swab is recommended and the technique is shown in Fig. II.1.★

★ Stratford, B. C., Rubbo, S. D., Christie, R. & Dixson, S. (1960) The treatment of the nasal carrier of *Staphylococcus aureus* with framycetin and other antibacterials. *Lancet*, **2**, 1125.

In some patients, particularly in babies, it is impossible to thread the swab deeply into the nose. In any case the procedure is mildly unpleasant and irritating, but is easily remedied by briskly rubbing the nose afterwards.

It is wise to request weekly routine nose and throat swabs from children and babies in hospital. Also the staff and patients in certain key areas must be regularly examined, e.g. in intensive care, cardiac surgery and neurosurgery departments. Similarly, compromised patients should be swabbed, e.g. patients with acute leukaemia or transplant recipients, or those on intermittent dialysis.

Nasal swabs are an important part of epidemic tracing whether the outbreak is due to *S. aureus*

Chapter 3
Throat Swabs

or to another pathogen, e.g. *Pseudomonas aeruginosa* or *Escherichia coli*.

The use of a tongue depressor with a good light from behind and over the left shoulder is most helpful in viewing the area to be swabbed. With the posterior pharyngeal wall visible, the swab is gently stroked over each tonsillar fossa (or tonsil) and then quickly streaked across the pharynx near the uvula (Fig. II.2). Disposable tongue depressors are now readily available and are better because one does not have to resterilize them.

Any exudate or membrane present is of the utmost diagnostic importance and should be swabbed off, or else lifted off with sterile forceps if it is adherent to the pharynx.

Some patients gag very easily, even when the tongue is merely touched with the depressor.

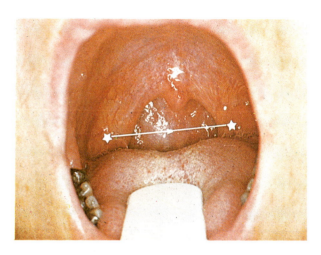

Fig. II.2. Areas to be swabbed when sampling the throat. See text, and note that it is unusual to obtain such a good view of the area to be swabbed, especially once the procedure is started, when speed in sampling is essential.

Fig. II.3. The correct method of holding a child for a throat swab. Note the restraining position of the attendant's arms.

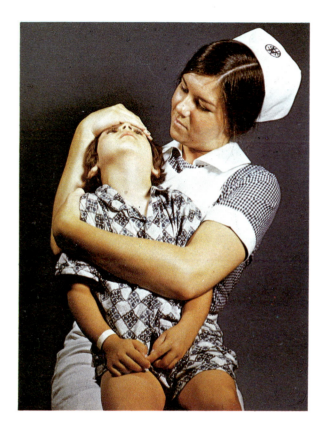

This must not prevent the operator from collecting the correct specimen, although some care may need to be taken.

Young children and babies normally give only one opportunity for taking a throat swab, and the moment they open their mouths to cry must be seized. Such young patients are best seated on someone's lap with chest and arms encircled by the assistant's left arm. With their right arm they hold the child's head firmly against their chest (Fig. II.3). The patient usually cries at this point.

If the attempt to take the specimen fails, the child often clamps its jaws firmly closed and only brute force can prise them open. It is better at this stage to lie him down with the body and head held firmly while another attempt is made to take the swab.

Throat swabs are required in cases of pharyngeal and tonsillar infections, or where diphtheria or contacts are suspected. They are also desirable from the key personnel and patients described in the previous chapter and also in times of epidemic sepsis. Many children's boarding hostels will not accept a child unless nose and throat swabs show the child is not carrying common communicable pathogens in his nose and throat.

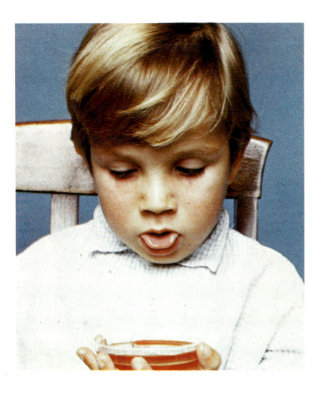

Fig. II.4. The use of a cough plate.
This child does not have whooping cough, but the picture illustrates the technique of the cough plate to be collected during a paroxysm caused by the disease.

Chapter 4
Cough Plates

Cough plates are seldom used now. Their importance lies in the identification of *Bordetella pertussis* when difficulty is experienced in obtaining sputum from a child.

The cough plate (Bordet-Gengou medium) is held 6 inches from the mouth during a typical paroxysm (Fig. II.4).

It is now thought more reliable to use a nasopharyngeal swab for diagnosis. The medium used for the cough plate contains penicillin to inhibit the majority of throat commensals thus permitting the growth of *B. pertussis*.

It should be noted that the child shown in the illustration is not suffering from whooping cough but is merely attempting to demonstrate the cough plate.

Chapter 5
Sputum

The nurse's urgent request to 'cough up a specimen' frequently results in hawked-up saliva or spittle being delivered to the laboratory as sputum. Such material is useless if one expects to detect microorganisms causing lower respiratory tract disease. Many of these are only feebly viable outside the chest. Therefore, sputum should reach the laboratory rapidly and such specimens should *not* be refrigerated.

A proper cough first thing in the morning is likely to produce sputum but sometimes the help of a chest physiotherapist is required to obtain the specimen. Clear containers are best used to allow the nurse or patient to see whether the specimen is truly sputum and also let the laboratory assess the specimen macroscopically

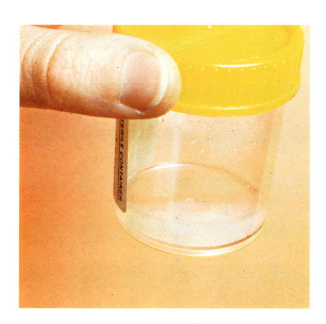

Fig. II.5. A typical specimen of saliva.
It should be easily noted by the nurse
that this is not a satisfactory specimen.

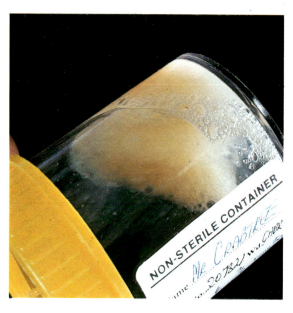

Fig. II.6. A sputum specimen. Again,
the clear container allows the collector
to see whether or not the specimen is
truly sputum.

(Figs. II.5 and II.6). The container lid should
be tightly fitting.

In the laboratory, ordinary handling of specimens of sputum often fails to detect a pathogen,
so specimens are best digested with either one
per cent sodium acetyl cysteine shaken for 15 min
or with one per cent buffered pancreatin which
is shaken for 5 min and then incubated at 37°C
for 30 min. These procedures produce a more
representative fraction of the specimen for
examination. They also allow a semi-quantitative
assessment of pathogens to decide whether infection or mere commensalism exists. Growth
overnight under CO_2 gives appreciably higher
yields of pathogens.*

* Burns, W. M., Devitt, Lorraine & Bryant, D. H. (1973) Why
do sputum cultures fail to yield pathogens? *Med. J. Aust.*, **2**, 768.

Details of the macroscopic presence of pus or
blood must be noted. Sputum examination for
tuberculosis is described in Chapter 12.

Some centres, notably the Mayo Clinic, will
not accept sputum as a specimen but insist on
trans-tracheal needle aspiration.

A new instrument the Colworth 'Stomacher'*
is now available which liquefies sputum and
other specimens in 30 sec.

This allows a quantitative count of organisms
to be made, and 10^8 is considered a significant
count, i.e. evidence of infection.

Counts between 10^4 and 10^7 are suspicious
and below 10^4 can be disregarded.

* Obtainable from A. J. Seward, London SE1 9U6.

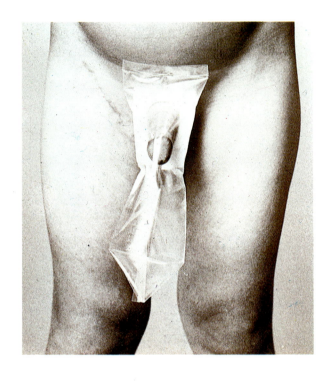

Fig. II.7. Neonatal urine collection apparatus. As can be seen, skin and anterior urethral contamination are unavoidable using such devices. This makes their urgent transport to the laboratory mandatory and their immediate processing necessary if results are to be meaningful.

Chapter 6
Urine

Urine is itself a good culture medium supporting the rapid multiplication of organisms at room temperature, so it is imperative that a specimen is examined within two hours of collection or else that it is refrigerated until examined.

Catheterization solely to obtain a bacteriological specimen is absolutely contraindicated. Eykyn and McFadyen* and others, recommend suprapubic puncture to obtain an uncontaminated specimen of bladder urine, but not all authorities would agree with this as a routine for obvious reasons. It is probably the only course

available if a patient is uncooperative or incontinent of urine.

Fig. II.7 illustrates an appliance used for the collection of urine in young children and neonates. Such collectors are almost calculated to give a contaminated specimen and here again bladder puncture may be justifiable.

The general opinion is that a *properly* collected midstream 'clean catch' urine is an adequate specimen. Provided the patient understands what is required most cooperate, at least in this country. It should be remembered that most people void better in private.

In the male, the prepuce is retracted and the glans is cleansed with soap and water. An anti-bacterial is unnecessary for this procedure. After

---

* Eykyn, Susanna J. & McFadyen, I. R. (1968) Suprapubic aspiration of urine in pregnancy. In *Urinary Tract Infection*, ed. F. O'Grady & W. Brumfitt. Oxford University Publications, p. 141.

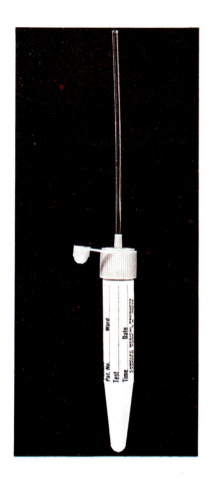

Fig. II.8. Sterile disposable urine collection centrifuge tube.* The capillary tube is dipped in the urine specimen, then the centrifuge tube is squeezed and a measured volume of urine is drawn up. The capillary tube is then broken off and the cap placed over the broken end of the tube. It is then ready to be sent to the laboratory.

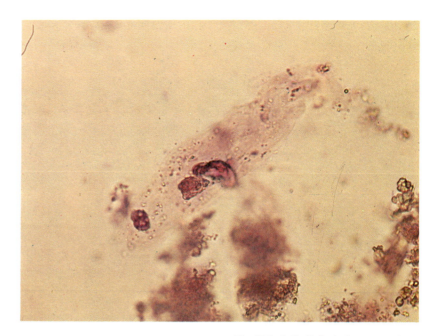

Fig. II.9. A Sedi-Stain® preparation of urine. This shows the cellular elements of urine well together with casts. The same elements can be seen without staining, but are less well marked. Crystals show up well. × 1326.

the first flow, about 50 ml of urine is collected in a screw-capped container or a sterile kidney dish. From this it can be taken up in a sterile disposable centrifuge tube for laboratory use (Fig. II.8).

In the female, the vulva is prepared in the same way, but swabbing *must* be from the front backwards to avoid anal contamination. The labia are separated by two fingers of the patient or a nurse while the specimen is passed and collected. It is usual to repeat a urine examination giving a colony count in excess of 100,000/ml before pronouncing infection present.*

The number and type of cells present can be reported per high power field, but more properly a cell count should be performed using a counting chamber such as a Fuchs Rosenthal.

A Sedi-Stain®† is a useful agent for demonstrating cells, casts or crystals that may be present in the spun deposit (Fig. II.9).

* Estimation of bacteria and white cells in the urine. *Association of Clinical Pathologists, Broadsheet* 80: August, 1973.

* Made by Camelec Medical Products, Camden Park, South Australia.
† Adams, Clay, *Sedi-Stain®*. Division of Becton, Dickinson & Co. Parsippany, N.J. 07054.

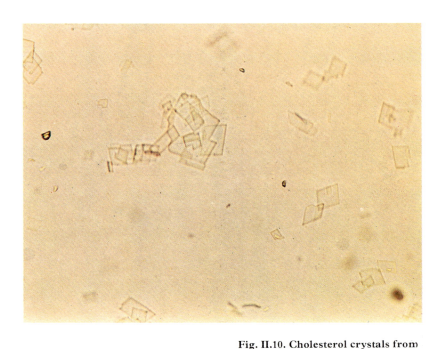

Fig. II.10. Cholesterol crystals from a pericardial effusion. Readers are referred to *Urine and the Urinary Sediment*, by R. W. Lippman, Charles C. Thomas, Springfield, Ill. (1972) 2nd ed. for the classical structure of crystals likely to be encountered in the microbiology laboratory. × 663.

Chapter 7
Pus and Wound Exudates

If swabs are to be used for obtaining and transporting the specimen, then it is best that they are serum-dipped. Ideally, a volume of pus in a sterile test tube or an excised piece of tissue (see Chapter 15) are better specimens. If ordinary swabs are employed and the inoculum is small, or the organism is fastidious, no growth may result, even though a prior Gram stain reveals the presence of microorganisms. In addition, the number of plates that may need to be used for complete identification of the organism limits the value of a single swab.

A quantity of pus in a test-tube allows macroscopic inspection which may give valuable clues both to the identification of the organism and the steps necessary to be taken for its growth,

e.g. the 'sulphur' granules of actinomycosis, or the greenish-blue coloured pus said to be characteristic of infection due to *Pseudomonas aeruginosa* (*pyocyanea*).

Under the heading of Pus and Wound Exudates, should properly come specimens from pericardial or pleural effusions. Here the prime cause may not be bacteriological but more likely viral or tuberculous. Equally, in joint effusions the laboratory may be expected to look for crystals. In the first two examples, the effusion may be massive in size, but it is preferable for the laboratory to be presented with a litre of fluid in a sterile jar for diagnosis rather than only 10 ml. Fig. II.10 shows cholesterol crystals from a pericardial effusion.

Chapter 8
Conjunctival Scrapings

The procedures required in dealing with specimens for anaerobic culture are dealt with in Chapter 17 and biopsy material in Chapter 15.

Vaginal swabs are dealt with more fully in Chapter 16. In general a blind vaginal swab (like a blind rectal swab) is an unsuitable specimen. In each instance the swab is best obtained under direct vision using a speculum or a proctoscope. Faecal specimens are detailed in Chapter 9.

Wound swabs are used normally to identify pyogenic organisms including anaerobic organisms (but see Chapter 17). Exudate specimens *may* grow similar organisms, but frequently the source of the exudate is either viral in origin (Chapter 19) or tuberculous (see Chapter 12).

Swabs are generally unsuitable for specimens from the conjunctival sac. First, if serum-dipped they are inclined to be rigid and hard after sterilization in a hot air oven for 1 hour at $160°C$, and second, if not dipped, small pieces of fibre may brush off in the sac and cause irritation.

The recommended method of obtaining a specimen from the eye is with a flamed and *cooled* small-diameter wire loop. The patient's head is tilted backwards in a comfortable but firm position with a good light. An assistant either pulls the lid downwards or upwards, whichever is appropriate, and a scraping is taken from the offending area using the loop, Fig. II.11. The contents of the loop are immediately streaked out onto chocolate agar (CA).

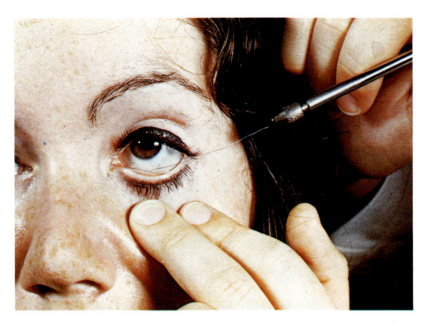

Fig. II.11. Method of obtaining a conjunctival specimen. A sterilized loop or a straight wire is best used for such specimens. In either instance it is better to take multiple scrapings if more than one plate needs to be inoculated.

A second scraping is used for a Gram stained specimen or Giemsa if inclusion body conjunctivitis is suspected.

Some ophthalmic surgeons prefer a preoperative report of any organisms in their patient's eyes two days before operation—the procedure is the same.

Chapter 9
Faeces

Rectal swabs, unless obtained under vision via a proctoscope, are much less satisfactory than a specimen of actual faeces. 'Blind' rectal swabs are generally quite useless from a diagnostic point of view as the natural inclination to tighten the sphincter ani makes most such swabs anal rather than rectal.

In general, faecal specimens are sent to the laboratory either to look for a bacterial cause of diarrhoea on the one hand or ova, cysts or parasites on the other. Much less frequently specimens of faeces are received in an endeavour to isolate viruses causing diarrhoea.

To search for faecal parasites, cysts or ova the specimen must be fresh and warm. Amoebae for example, quickly lose their characteristic morphology and motility if left standing at room temperature.

For bacteriological diagnosis, time is not so critical, but if the delay in examination extends over 12 hours, the faeces should be added to an equal volume of buffered glycerol saline and the two well mixed. Viral transport medium is discussed in Chapter 19.

Apart from the more usual bacteriological causes of infective diarrhoea such as *Salmonella* and *Shigella spp.* it is now well-established practice to search for enteropathogenic *Escherichia coli* not only in infants but also in the elderly, and perhaps there is a case for this investigation at any age.

The presence of purulent ulcers in the rectum or sigmoid colon suggests amoebiasis, and is a special case dealt with under the investigation of rectal ulcers in Chapter 15. Chronic dysentery often presents a similar morphological picture but it is important to note that the laboratory is in a position to clarify the diagnosis.

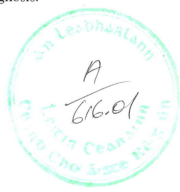

Chapter 10
Cerebrospinal Fluid

A lumbar puncture is no light matter for a patient and the specimen is important, therefore the laboratory should be warned that one is expected. The microscopic examination of CSF for a cell count and a Gram stain for organisms should be performed within half an hour of its being taken. After about an hour or more the cells disintegrate if left at room temperature or in the refrigerator and thus the immediate diagnostic significance of the lumbar tap may be lost.

The specimen should be taken into a sterile glass test-tube or better, a centrifuge tube, where the macroscopic appearance can be easily noted, and in fact the specimen is then ready to be centrifuged, thus reducing the chance of laboratory contamination.

In acute pyogenic meningitis the specimen is usually turbid, but varies from clear to frankly purulent. In aseptic or viral meningitis the fluid is often clear as is frequently the case when the meningitis is tuberculous in origin or due to *Cryptococcus neoformans*, or in the case of early pyogenic meningitis.

As meningitis is a medical emergency, the total and differential white cell count, combined with the findings obtained from Gram or Zeihl-Neelsen stains, or India ink preparations are the first guide to immediate therapy; so these must be performed with the utmost care and accuracy. A 'bloody' tap is not infrequent and quite unavoidable when it happens, but this should not preclude the above tests being easily per-

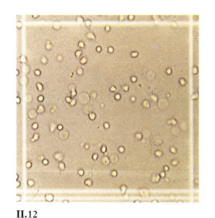
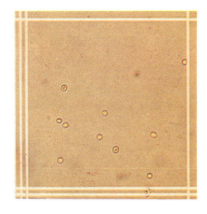

II.12

Fig. II.12A. Acute pyogenic meningitis. In a Fuchs Rosenthal counting chamber the *uncentrifuged* deposit is counted and the white cell numbers are differentiated for the clinician. Note that in this preparation polymorphonuclear leucocytes predominate. × 282.

Fig. II.12B. Chronic meningitis due to Cryptococcus neoformans. The picture in the counting chamber is one of essential lymphocytosis. Without special staining techniques *C. neoformans* cells resemble lymphocytes. × 282.

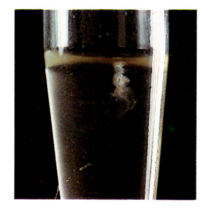

Fig. II.13. 'Spider web' coagulum in CSF.

formed by dilution using white cell diluting fluid.* Fig. II.12A shows the picture in a Fuchs Rosenthal counting chamber of a case of acute pyogenic meningitis, and Fig. II.12B the situation in a case of meningitis due to *C. neoformans.*

Most large hospitals take the lumbar puncture specimen into two tubes—the second being for biochemical evaluation. If only one tube is obtained, it is essential that the microbiology laboratory has first claim on it—not only to work with the uncontaminated and fresh specimen, but also because its findings are of more urgent importance than are the (somewhat irregular) biochemical results in cases of meningitis which frequently are not of specific diagnostic importance.*

Some authorities still recommend leaving a potentially tuberculosis specimen to stand for an hour until a characteristic 'spider web' coagulum forms (Fig. II.13). From this clot, if it forms, organisms are readily demonstrated. This method is better used later in the disease because it is often not found early. It can indeed be used as a measure of progress of chemotherapy.

The presence of polymorphs in the CSF in the absence of bacteria should suggest primary

---

* WHITE CELL DILUTING FLUID

Glacial acetic acid	1.5 ml
1 % aqueous solution of gentian violet	1.0 ml
Distilled water	98 ml

* Anderson, Kevin F. (1973) Diagnosis and treatment of meningitis. *Med. J. Aust.,* **1**, 897.

amoebic meningo-encephalitis caused by the free-living amoeba *Naegleria fowleri* which is easily seen under phase microscopy when a fresh specimen is examined.

Chapter 11
Blood Cultures

Blood cultures are performed in an endeavour to grow microorganisms from the blood of patients suffering from septicaemia, bacterial endocarditis, bacteraemia or typhoid fever. Because of the coarse nature of specimen collection, blood culture bottles are often contaminated with skin commensals, thus making early interpretation of the results difficult for the clinician. For this reason extreme care must be exercised in the performance of venepuncture and the transfer of the blood to the blood culture bottles, also in changing syringes should this prove necessary.

Most laboratories use two bottles, one for aerobic culture (sometimes including an agar slope for easy subculture) and the second for anaerobic culture; some use a third bottle with added sucrose to produce a hypertonic medium for the culture of L-forms or protoplasts. Others use special media for fungi and also culture under CO_2.

In either instance the amount of blood drawn is critical as the number of organisms available for growth depends on the inoculum size—in this case the volume of blood taken. It is, therefore, important to take as much blood as is possible at the time; but it must be remembered that changing syringes is another opportunity for contamination unless done with some expertise.

Many clinicians, convinced of the diagnosis of septicaemia, request serial blood cultures because of the importance of early diagnosis and the urgency of this demands that the laboratory personnel inspect blood culture bottles at least once daily for evidence of turbidity or growth.

Some organisms grow rapidly, such as *S. aureus*, other quick multipliers such as *P. aeruginosa* discolour and lyse the blood and produce a characteristic pellicle; these facts taken in conjunction with a Gram stain, allow a presumptive diagnosis to be made quite early in the course of the disease.

Because of the risk of contamination from the skin either of the patient or the operator, a full aseptic ritual should be employed during venepuncture in these cases. The operator should be masked and gowned and wear sterile gloves, preferably disposable. The patient's skin in the

Fig. II.14. The technique of antecubital venepuncture. After the arm has been prepared (see text), a tourniquet applied, the operator, gowned and gloved takes blood from the vein.

Fig. II.15. Articles required for blood culture.
1 At least two 20 ml syringes (preferably disposable).
2 At least two guage 19 disposable needles.
3 Tourniquet.
4 Drapes.
5 Alcoholic chlorhexidine pressure pack or similar skin disinfectant.
6 Swabs.
7 Aerobic blood culture bottle. (left)
8 L-form blood culture bottle. (middle)
9 Anaerobic blood culture bottle. (right)
10 The operator needs to be scrubbed, gowned, masked, etc. (gloves, mask)

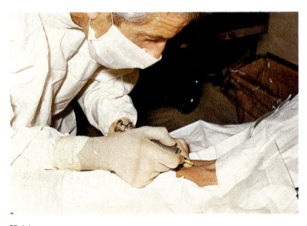

II.14

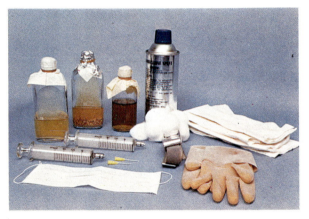

II.15

area of venepuncture should be washed thoroughly with an inert soap and water, dried with a sterile towel, and then carefully disinfected with alcoholic chlorhexidine (Hibitane®) or Povidone-iodine® after a tourniquet has been applied.

The area is draped as for operation and the appropriate amount(s) of blood taken in 20 ml disposable syringes and carefully transferred into the blood culture bottles. The latter should be well labelled with name, date, time, etc. and should be individually distinctive so that the operator does not accidentally use say, two 'aerobic' bottles.

Some clinicians take blood in the case of a suspected Gram negative septicaemia when the

temperature is in the trough, on the ascent and at the peak. The rationale behind taking blood when the temperature is low is that this is the likely time that organisms are dividing and there is a stronger possibility of a positive result.

The technique of antecubital venepuncture together with the materials for blood culture used in this hospital are shown in Figs. II.14 and II.15.

Clot culture is explained in Chapter 13—Enteric Fevers.

Chapter 12
Tuberculosis

Although tuberculosis is much less common than it was in Western countries it is still an important differential diagnosis and considerable care needs to be taken in examination of specimens to avoid missing the diagnosis. It is customary to request specimens of sputum or urine for the detection of tuberculosis on three successive mornings. This does not apply to pleural fluid or CSF, but both of these should be treated with sterile sodium citrate to prevent clotting. However, some authorities still prefer to culture the 'spider web' clot which occurs late in a tuberculous CSF (see Fig. II.13).

1 Sputum and Bronchial Washings

As with other specimens of sputum it is imperative that the sample should be truly sputum and not saliva. On reaching the laboratory, the specimen is digested and shaken with an equal volume of one per cent sodium acetyl cysteine or one per cent buffered pancreatin as in Chapter 5. These agents liquefy the sputum which is then treated with 15 per cent trisodium phosphate $(Na_3PO_412H_2O)^\star$ for 2–3 hours at $37^\circ C$ to destroy bacteria other than *Mycobacterium tuberculosis*. It is then spun down for 15 minutes to concentrate any *M. tuberculosis* into a small

$\star$ *Procedures for the Laboratory Diagnosis of Mycobacterial Infection* (1973), 4th ed. Australian Government Publishing Service, Canberra.

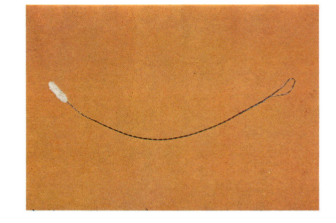

Fig. II.16. Laryngeal swab. The long and curved nature of the swab allows it to be passed to the vocal cords, this induces coughing and any bronchial secretions are therefore sampled.

volume. Two ml of sterile saline are added to the sediment which is then cultured on Lowenstein-Jensen slopes. Zeihl-Neelsen staining can be performed from the original specimen or the sediment. An Auramine-Rhodamine stain is much quicker if a fluorescent microscope is available and the user experienced; but a ZN re-stain must always be performed on a supposedly positive AR to prove the presence of acid-fast bacilli.

LJ slopes are examined weekly for the presence of growth which must then be proved to be *M. tuberculosis*. If there is no growth after 9 weeks the specimens are discarded.

Guinea pig inoculation is not used so commonly now as formerly but must be performed

if Koch's postulates are to be satisfied. Treatment of *bronchial washings* is the same as for sputum.

2   Laryngeal Swab

These swabs (Fig. II.16) are not often used now. Their major value lies in obtaining material from the larynx for culture when sputum is absent or impossible to collect, e.g. in small children. In the laboratory the same procedure of digestion with a solution of trisodium phosphate and incubation at 37°C is carried out. The swab is removed and placed in fluid which is centrifuged, the supernatant is then decanted and the deposit is inoculated onto two LJ slopes. This is repeated on three successive mornings.

3 Gastric Lavage

In patients with no sputum or those who swallow their sputum, stomach contents in the fasting state may be aspirated via a Ryle's tube on three successive mornings after 20 ml of sterile saline has been passed down the tube. The aspirate is taken into a screw-capped bottle containing trisodium phosphate crystals and the same procedure is carried out as with sputum above. Although the tubercle bacillus is hardy it is wise to perform gastric lavage no earlier than an hour before the laboratory commences work in the morning even if this means fasting the patient for another hour or two. This technique is more successful than the use of a laryngeal swab.

4 Urine

Three complete early morning specimens are carefully collected and sent immediately to the laboratory or else refrigerated. The specimen is centrifuged and treated in the same way as sputum. Smears are made from the deposit. It is routine to perform a colony count in the normal way as the presence of another bacterial infection indicates a need for treatment before *M. tuberculosis* can be looked for because it is easily overgrown by other microorganisms, particularly those which are Gram negative.

5 Aspirate Fluids

These may be pleural, pericardial, ascitic or synovial. These specimens should be taken into sterile sodium citrate or a sterile heparinized tube or container. Subsequent handling is the same as for urine, but if the specimen is not sterile it requires overnight treatment with trisodium phosphate at 37°C.

6 Pus or Bone Marrow

Pus always requires overnight incubation treatment with trisodium phosphate, whereas bone marrow aspirate usually does not. Laboratory procedure is the same as for urine.

7 Tissue Biopsies

Some specimens of tissue, or more often excised lymph nodes, are usually presumed to be uncontaminated. It is normal practice to share the specimen with the anatomical pathologists for histological section. The specimen should be divided aseptically in the microbiology laboratory—in this way it does not arrive in formalin for culture! The specimen is then homogenized under sterile conditions using saline in a mechanical blender. A sterility check on BA is performed overnight. If this is positive the homogenate is digested in the normal way. If it is sterile, the homogenate can then be inoculated onto LJ medium. ZN or AR stains are then performed on the homogenate.

Note : It is vital that a safety cabinet be used for processing specimens for tuberculosis—also the operator must wear protective clothing, a mask and disposable gloves. The cabinet should be well exhausted to a safe spot high in the outside air.

Chapter 13
Enteric Fevers

The enteric fevers include diseases caused by *Salmonella typhi* and the agents causing paratyphoid fever. The latter are both less common and less important sources of disease in Western countries, but the disease caused is clinically similar to typhoid fever.

Laboratory diagnosis of *S. typhi* infection depends on two things; first, the isolation from the body and identification of the causative organism, and second, evidence of its presence in the body by the Widal agglutination test. Table II.1 shows the best times for taking the appropriate specimens in salmonellosis.

Table II.1 Optimal times for collecting specimens in Salmonella infections.

Time	Specimen	
7–10 days incubation		
1–10 days post incubation	Blood Clot culture Widal	} Bile-salt broth
10–13 days	Bone marrow	Bile-salt broth
7–14 days post incubation	Stool	(May be positive)
7–21 days *et seq.*	Urine	(May be positive)
	Carrier state (days, months or years) (Stool and urine may be intermittently positive)	

N.B. *S. typhimurium* infections are generally much quicker in all stages.

1 Blood Culture

In the first 7–10 days of the disease, positive blood culture is the most conclusive diagnostic method. This can also be used if the patient is considered to have relapsed. No matter which culture medium is normally employed for blood culture, it is essential for the diagnosis of enteric fever that the medium contain bile salts, e.g. 0.5 per cent sodium taurocholate.

2 Clot Culture

Many authorities regard clot culture at least equally important as blood cultures in the diagnosis of enteric fever. Here the blood is allowed to clot and the supernatant serum removed. The clot is added aseptically to bile-salt broth containing streptokinase which rapidly lyses the clot liberating any organisms present. Subsequent steps are the same as for blood culture.

After 7–10 days of illness the likelihood of finding the microorganisms in the blood progressively lessens. Some laboratories perform *bone marrow culture* which is said to remain positive for a day or two after antibiotic therapy is begun, but this is of doubtful value as a diagnostic aid.

3 Urine Culture

Urine culture may be positive in the second week of the disease but needs to be performed daily. Rarely, urine specimens may reveal the causative organisms at other times—even in the carrier state. In these circumstances it is important that care is taken in the collection of the specimens to avoid faecal contamination thus erroneously labelling a faecal carrier a urine carrier.

Bacilluria is frequently intermittent and the best specimen is the entire early morning one. This is centrifuged and several loopfuls of the sediment are used as the inoculum.

4 Faecal Culture

The organisms causing enteric fever are easily isolated from the faeces throughout the disease, but particularly in the second and third weeks provided the correct selective media are used. As with any specimen, the more that are examined the more likely it is that a positive result will be obtained. Because of the contagious nature of these diseases, if they are suspected by the clinician the laboratory must process as many specimens as are required to prove the diagnosis or otherwise.

5 Bile Culture

Aspirate from the duodenum can be obtained via a Ryle's tube. This test needs to be positive in carriers before a cholecystectomy can be expected to cure the carrier state. It should be noted that in many countries a positive culture constitutes a notifiable disease.

Chapter 14
Leptospirosis

The best known form of leptospirosis is Weil's disease, but subclinical and less severe infection is known to be much more common and is best proved by serology (Chapter 40).

In the acute disease, examination of a blood film directly using dark-ground illumination or after staining by Giemsa may show the characteristic leptospira.

Blood Culture

This can be performed using a variety of media. It is suggested that the most reliable is sterile 10 per cent inactivated rabbit serum employing a large inoculum of blood. Incubation is at 37°C and samples are examined twice a week under dark-ground illumination for up to 4 weeks. If growth is observed the incubation temperature should be changed to 30°C.

Animal Inoculation

Hamsters or guinea pigs are the most sensitive diagnostic tools. Fresh plasma or urine is inoculated intraperitoneally. After a matter of only a few days spirochaetes can be found in the peritoneal exudate. Cardiac puncture is then performed to obtain blood from the animal for culture.

In the case of virulent organisms, in 4–6 days the animal fails to thrive and its coat roughens. Jaundice occurs two or three days later and the animal dies on the 8–14th day. Haemorrhagic lesions are found in many organs and in these

Chapter 15
Specimens from Other Infections

the microorganism abounds. Full and sterile precautions must be taken in the handling and autopsy of such animals.

The microbiology laboratory is not infrequently called upon to determine whether a variety of other specimens are infected, or alternatively, whether certain items for human use are sterile. Routine sterilization methods are not a proper subject for this book and many reliable texts are available.★

Some of the more common specimens sent to the laboratory for processing are detailed below.

1 Biopsy Specimens

These are taken in the operating theatre using a

★ Rubbo, S. D. & Gardner, Joan F. (1977) *A Review of Sterilization and Disinfection*, 2nd ed. Lloyd-Luke (Medical Books) Ltd., London.

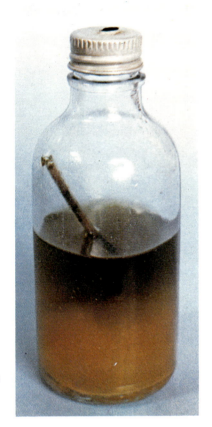

Fig. II.17. Culture of catheter tip.
Note the catheter tip in Brewer's thioglycollate broth. Where turbidity is seen in the brown bottom half it indicates growth in the anaerobic medium.

full aseptic ritual and can be presumed not contaminated if placed immediately in a sterile container. They should be transferred to the laboratory with all speed for processing. Any delay in transport to the laboratory only reduces the chance of isolating pathogens so surgeons and theatre staff should be aware of this fact. To save accidental immersion in formalin it is better to send the specimen 'dry' and not insist on immersion in sterile saline.

Such specimens of tissue are finely ground in a sterile homogenizer in a safety cabinet, and then examined and plated out in the appropriate manner. The Colwell 'Stomacher' is the best homogenizer, see p. 13.

2 Catheters

The tips of intravenous, cardiac and even urinary catheters are sometimes sent for culture. These are best cultured in Brewer's thioglycollate broth (Fig. II.17).

3 Intravenous Fluids

It is mandatory in view of recent happenings, to routinely 'batch test' intravenous fluids for sterility. The sample is withdrawn by perforating the cap. Small samples of fluid are best tested in thioglycollate broth. With larger volumes it is preferable to draw the entire solution through a Millipore® filter (pore size $0.20\ \mu$) with no added

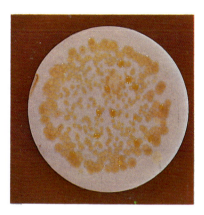

Fig. II.18. Growth on a millipore filter disc. Note the two different types of colonies which have grown on the upper surface of the filter paper disc. If any growth occurs following filtration of a representative number of bottles of solution, then the whole batch of solutions must be discarded.

pressure or vacuum. The entire filter is carefully removed and incubated on B.A. at 30°C for 10 days. Colonies, if contamination is present, grow on the upper surface of the filter (Fig. II.18).

4   Rectal or Sigmoid Ulcer Specimens

Depending on the clinical picture, rectal or sigmoid ulcers may suggest a diagnosis of amoebiasis or ulcerative colitis. In either event a careful scraping must be taken under direct vision through a sigmoidoscope and transferred immediately to a glass slide. This must be examined as a wet preparation *as soon as possible* to determine the presence or absence of vegetative amoebae if a strong clinical suspicion exists

(see Chapter 56). Other scrapings can be examined with more leisure to determine the bacteriological content.

5   Crystals

The laboratory may be asked to decide the correct nature of crystals in a specimen, say from a joint or a urinary sediment. Excellent examples of such findings are in most biochemistry texts, but the urinary sediment is well described by Lippman.*

---

* Lippman, R. W. & Thomas, Charles (1972) *Urine and Urinary Sediment*, Springfield, Illinois, U.S.A.

Chapter 16
Venereal Disease

Gloves and gown must be worn when collecting specimens from a patient suspected of having venereal disease because *Treponena pallidum* can pass through the intact skin.

A number of attitudes in present day sexual practice determine the type of specimens that need to be taken for diagnosis; amongst these are homosexual relationships, fellatio and a propensity for the gonococcus to survive only in the rectum in a significant number of females suffering from the chronic form of the disease. It should be stressed that in the female the gonococcus may produce remarkably few symptoms or signs, and it has recently been suggested that in the male the same circumstances may prevail.

1 Gonorrhoea

This disease is increasing in both sexes universally; although the incidence of syphilis is also increasing, the rate is not so fast as gonorrhoea and also in syphilis most of the increase appears to be in male homosexuals.

Swabs to isolate the gonococcus should be taken under direct vision, e.g. the urethra is easily seen in both sexes, a proper cervical swab requires a vaginal speculum, a rectal swab should be taken through a proctoscope, and finally pharyngeal swabs are taken under full observation (see Fig. II.2).

The swabs required in suspect cases of gonorrhoea whether acute or chronic are listed in

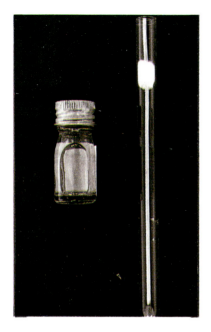

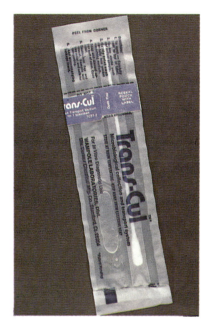

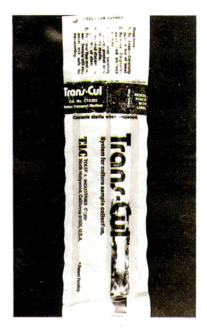

Fig. II.19. Conventional Stuart swab kit. This type of swab kit is normally made up by the hospital media room or supplied by area Public Health Authorities. Note the charcoal tipped swab. After taking the specimen the swab is broken off in the medium and the screw cap closed tightly. Organisms retain viability in this medium for 48–72 hours.

Fig. II.20. Trans-Cul® transport medium. In this photograph the kit is shown unused, with the swab stick on one side and the Stuart's medium on the other.

Fig. II.21. Used Trans-Cul® transport medium. This photograph shows the used swab placed in the Amies charcoal transport medium. The top of the plastic has not been folded down as would be required once the specimen was taken in practice.

Table II.2. It should be remembered that symptoms and signs may be minimal except in the patient with flagrant urethritis.

'Blind' vaginal swabs are unsuitable for diagnosis. Also, unless swabs can be examined within half an hour of collection they must be placed in Stuart's or Amies Transport Medium.★ Acceptable variations of this are shown in Figs. II.19, II.20, and II.21. The gonococcal complement fixation text is discussed in Chapter 33.

★ Trans-Cul® swab kits are supplied by T.I.C.—Toluca Industries Corporation, North Hollywood, Calif. 91605 U.S.A. The one pictured is Amies Transport Medium, but they also supply, in similar form, Stuart's Transport Medium. In this hospital, for general diagnosis, we have found the Amies Transport Medium to be the better of the two.

Table II.2 Routine swabs required for the diagnosis of gonorrhoea.

Swab	Male	Female
Pharyngeal	+	+
Rectal	+	+
Urethral	+	+
Cervical	−	+

It should be remembered that *Neisseria gonorrhoeae* occasionally invades the blood stream and may produce lesions at a distance, e.g. joints, tendon sheaths, heart valves, skin and meninges. Nowadays, one rarely sees conjunctivitis due to this organism in infants, but vulvo-vaginitis in young girls still occurs. Appropriate specimens *v.s.* need to be taken from such lesions.

2 Syphilis

Dark-ground illumination is employed to demonstrate spirochaetes in wet preparations made from scrapings using a sterile loop to obtain the specimen from a possible primary chancre after prior cleansing with sterile saline (not an antibacterial). Chancres can occur anywhere on the body, but commonly are seen on the genital area or around the anus. The same type of examination is positive for fluid removed from a papule of the secondary rash of syphilis. One must stress again the high infectivity of these lesions and the need for the operator to take suitable precautions when obtaining specimens.

Syphilis serology is discussed in detail in Chapter 39. It should also be remembered that acute gonorrhoea and primary syphilis may coexist and appropriate specimens especially blood, should be taken at regular intervals to exclude syphilis. Also prior treatment of acute gonorrhoea with any antibiotic, or suboptimal doses of penicillin may mask the development of primary syphilis when a patient is being examined for what appears to be an uncomplicated case of gonorrhoea.

3 Granuloma Inguinale

The biological characteristics of the causative organism are still doubtful, but the disease is observed in tropical and subtropical countries.

The initial lesion is normally genital. The organism is a small $(1-2\,\mu)$ pleomorphic Gram negative bacillus which grows only on yolk sac culture. Blood should be taken for complement fixation testing.

4 Lymphogranuloma Venereum

This is not the same as the former disease. After an incubation period of 1 to 3 weeks a primary sore appears on the genitalia. It becomes vesicular and then ulcerates. The causative virus then spreads to involve the regional lymph nodes which may suppurate. The virus belongs to the psittacosis group and grows abundantly in the yolk sac of developing chick embryos. Aspirated pus from a bubo may be used for virus cultivation. Blood may be taken for the complement fixation test and a skin test (the Frei test) is available.

Chapter 17
Specimens for Anaerobic Culture

Little extra trouble is required to put up specimens for anaerobic as well as aerobic culture. The real problem arises when one asks 'is this good enough?'

A strong body of opinion currently holds the view that clinicians should *request* anaerobic culture whenever the possibility of such an infection exists. One excludes *Clostridium welchii (perfringens)* from this discussion where both the clinician and the microbiologist are in complete accord so far as the specimens which are required to make a diagnosis.

It is obviously true that in the past *Bacteroides spp.* and other fastidious anaerobes have been missed in laboratory diagnosis, mainly because they have not been looked for. However, the possibility of finding such anaerobes depends first, on the correct specimen being sent, second, the time delay in the taking of the specimen and its being processed in the laboratory, third, that the specimen is sent in an appropriate container for anaerobic culture, and finally the requirement that the laboratory is notified so that they are ready to receive the specimen within 10 minutes of its being taken.

It should be noted that *swabs are quite unsuitable* for anaerobic culture. This applies even to specimens where less fastidious anaerobes such as *C. welchii* are concerned. Wherever possible a volume of pus or a portion of excised tissue is much more likely to result in a positive diagnosis.

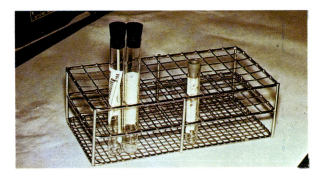

Fig. II.22. 'Gassed out' tubes. This
tube, as the name suggests, is evacuated,
so any fluid, e.g. pus, put into it via a
syringe should NOT include any air.
Such tubes (Vacutainer®) are supplied by
Becton-Dickinson and Co.

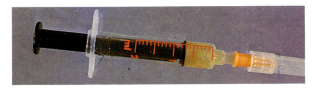

Fig. II.23. 'Closed syringe' technique
for an anaerobic specimen. The
syringe has been used to aspirate the
pus. A stopper covers the needle and as
no air is present it provides completely
anaerobic conditions for transfer of the
specimen to the laboratory.

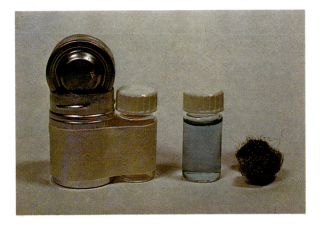

Fig. II.24. Copper sulphate transport
system. An ordinary 35 mm film
container is sterilized in the hot air oven.
The specimen is then placed in it, at the
same time the copper sulphate solution
and 'steel' wool is used to produce
anaerobic conditions.

The methods of transporting specimens from
the patient to the laboratory are as follows:

1 'Gassed Out' Tubes

These are evacuated tubes containing no air and
thus suitable for transport of fluid specimens
(Fig. II.22).

2 'Closed Syringes'

An ordinary syringe can be used to aspirate
fluid or pus and then the needle cover is placed
over the end of the needle. The whole syringe
can then be taken to the laboratory as the sterile
specimen container (Fig. II.23).

3 Copper Sulphate Transport System

This system, illustrated in Fig. II.24 employs
copper sulphate to provide anaerobic conditions
for a specimen in the container shown. Any
hospital can make its own system using 35 mm
film containers with a rubber stopper, 'steel'
(iron) wool and copper sulphate (10 per cent)
solution.

4 Other Methods

Specimens may also be transported in commercially available reduced transport medium,
or in anaerobic blood culture medium.

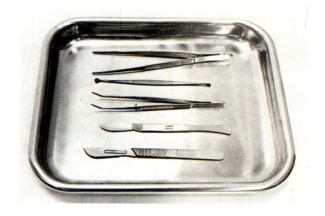

Fig. II.25. Instruments required to obtain a specimen for mycology.
Such a tray may be sterilized *in toto* or each instrument can be separately sterilized in an appropriate container.
1 Flat-headed forceps.
2 Curette.
3 Fine, curved, pointed dental forceps.
4 Scalpel knife.
5 Scalpel handle with No. 22 surgical blade.

Chapter 18
Specimens for Mycological Examination

A minimum number of instruments required to take mycology specimens is shown in Fig. II.25. As with any other microbiological technique, the demonstration of fungi depends on the calibre and correctness of the specimen taken for/or in the laboratory.

Fragments of skin obtained by scraping, specimens of hair or nail cuttings must be deliberately taken into a sterile Petri dish and then prepared for examination. These are usually 'cleared', i.e. made transparent, so that any fungal hyphae may be visible. Depending on the specimen, it must be digested with 10 per cent potassium hydroxide (KOH) to dissolve the keratin so that the fungi are made readily visible by staining, e.g. with lactophenol blue, and also the specimen is

ready for culture. Gram staining may also be used in the diagnosis of actinomycotic infections. Giemsa stain is particularly useful for *Malassezia furfur*.

In the case of Tinea capitis, caused by *Microsporum canis, M. audouinii*, and *T. schoenleinii*, infected hairs fluoresce under a Wood's lamp, which should be a standard part of the equipment of a laboratory. The patient can be examined using the lamp and then appropriate specimens taken for staining and culture.

India-ink preparations are used to show the characteristic capsule of *Cryptococcus neoformans* on primary examination, e.g. in CSF.

It should be remembered that identification of fungi according to their cultural characteristics

Chapter 19
Specimens for Viral Studies

requires the examination of both the agar and bottom surfaces of the plate, see Section IV.

Throat and nasal washings, naso-pharyngeal swabs, faeces, urine, CSF and vesicle fluids all serve as suitable sources of material for virus isolation from clinical cases. Serum is used for serological investigations (Chapter 64), but whole blood is rarely employed. Specimens are placed in viral transport medium (*v.i.*) and for short distances should be kept in wet ice. For longer distances dry ice is required, an exception here is the respiratory syncytial virus which is rapidly inactivated by freezing and thawing. The stages of clinical illness most favourable for virus isolation are indicated in Table II.3.

Table II.3. Relationship between the stage of clinical illness to the time most suitable for virus isolation.

Stage of illness	Likelihood of virus isolation
Incubation	− generally, occasionally + in blood
Prodrome	+
Onset	+ + +
Acute	+ + +
Recovery	+ +
Convalescence	− generally, an obvious exception are the enteroviruses.

Sero-Diagnosis

Antibodies to a particular infecting virus are usually not detectable until the onset of clinical symptoms but reach their maximum titre between 1 and 2 weeks later. For a positive serological diagnosis, it is necessary to observe a significant rise in titre (generally fourfold) between the acute and convalescent stages of the disease. See Chapter 64.

Transport Media

The specimen or swab is suspended in a suitable medium, which usually consists of an isotonic salt solution containing gelatin or bovine albumin (0.2–0.5 per cent), antibiotics and a suitable pH indicator, normally phenol red. Antibiotics used include penicillin (100 μg/ml) and/or streptomycin (100 μg/ml), but with faecal specimens amphotericin B (2.5 μg/ml) or nystatin (40 μg/ml) are also included to inhibit either yeast or fungal growth.

A small amount of protein is included to protect any virus present in the specimen from thermal inactivation. Inactivation is also brought about by extremes of pH and the indicator is included to determine whether such losses are likely to have occurred.

Types of Specimens Required for Virus Isolation

A summary of the broad clinical features of viral diseases and the types of specimens required for the isolation of individual viruses is given in Table II.4.

Preparation of Specimens for Attempted Virus Isolation

(a) STERILE SPECIMENS

Specimens such as CSF, white blood cells, plasma or urine may be inoculated directly into cell culture or embryonated eggs as required, without the addition of antibiotics.

(b) TISSUE SPECIMENS

Where a tissue sample is provided, it is necessary to prepare a 10 per cent homogenate in transport medium using a mechanical blender. Cell debris should then be removed by centrifuging at 1000–2000 g for 10–15 minutes and penicillin and streptomycin (at five times the concentration used in transport medium) added to the supernate. After leaving at 4°C for 1 hour, aliquots of the treated supernatant are then inoculated into cell cultures, embryonated eggs, or other hosts.

Table II.4. Specimens for virus isolation.

Clinical Manifestation of Infection	Possible Aetiological Agent	Specimen Material	
		Clinical	Autopsy.
Upper respiratory tract infection	Rhino Influenza Parainfluenza Corona	Throat swab or Nasal washings	—
	Adeno Coxsackie Echo Respiratory syncitial	Throat swab or Faeces	—
Lower respiratory tract infection	Influenza Adeno Parainfluenza Rhino Mycoplasma pneumoniae	Throat washings	Lung, Tracheal swab.
Vesicular lesions of skin and mucous membranes	Smallpox and vaccinia Herpes simplex Varicella/zoster Coxsackie	Vesicle fluid Throat swab Faeces	Liver, spleen, lung, vesicle fluid.
Skin rashes	Measles Rubella Some Arbo	Throat washings or nasal swab, and blood.	—
	Coxsackie Echo	Throat washings or swab, faeces.	—
C.N.S. infections	Coxsackie Echo Polio	Faeces, CSF Throat swab	Brain, spinal cord, and intestinal contents.
	Herpex simplex	Throat washings or swab.	Brain tissue.
	Rabies	Saliva.	Brain tissue.
	Mumps	Throat washings, CSF and urine.	—
	Some Arthropod-borne	Throat swabs, CSF.	Brain tissue
Arthropod-borne Infections	Various members of the Alpha- Flavi- Arena and Bunyamwera groups.	Blood and CSF.	Brain tissue.
Congenital infections	Cytomegalo	Urine and throat swab.	Kidney, lung, and other tissues.
	Rubella	Nasal swab, urine.	Lymph nodes, lung, spleen and other tissues. Also the fetus and placenta.
Hepatitis A	Unclassified	*Blood, faeces	Liver
Hepatitis B	Unclassified	Blood, faeces, urine.	Liver.

* Not generally available.

(c) THROAT AND NASAL WASHINGS, THROAT SWABS

Suspensions of throat washings are prepared with an equal volume of transport medium, while fluid from the swabs is expressed into 1–2 ml of the same medium. Penicillin, streptomycin, amphotericin B or nystatin are added at 10 times their normal concentration and the suspension is allowed to stand at 4°C for 1 hour before being used to inoculate cell cultures or embryonated eggs.

(d) FAECAL AND HEAVILY CONTAMINATED SPECIMENS

One method is where a 10 per cent suspension is prepared in transport medium in a screw-capped jar containing glass beads; the specimen is then emulsified by vigorous shaking. If necessary it may be further broken up in a mechanical blender. The suspension should then be clarified by centrifuging at 5000 g for 10–15 minutes and the supernatant filtered through a layer of sterile gauze and further centrifuged in an ultracentrifuge at 8000 g for 1 hour.

Penicillin, streptomycin and amphotericin B should then be added to the second supernate at 25 times their normal concentration and the mixture kept at 4°C for 1 hour before being used for inoculation. The fluid from faecal swabs is expressed into 1–2 ml transport medium and ultracentrifuged and treated with antibiotics before being used for inoculation.

SECTION III
SYSTEMATIC
BACTERIOLOGY

Introduction

Bacteria are microscopic organisms having a primitive simple form of cellular organization. Although generally unicellular, they grow in pairs (diplococci), clusters (staphylococci), chains (streptococci) or as rods (bacilli). The higher bacteria (*Actinomyces*) have filaments. Bacterial cells are smaller than those of protozoa or fungi. They possess a relatively rigid cell wall which maintains their characteristic shape, e.g. spherical (coccus), rod-shaped (bacillus), comma-shaped (vibrio), spiral (spirillum and sphirochaete) or else filamentous forms.

Bacteria can be classified by Gram staining although certain special stains are also required, e.g. Ziehl-Neelsen for *Mycobacterium tuberculosis*, and Albert's stain can be used for the

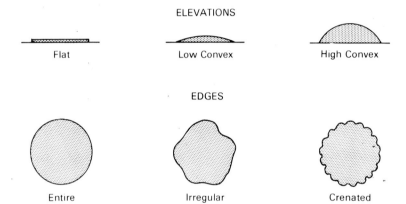

ELEVATIONS AND EDGES OF COMMON TYPES OF COLONIES

ELEVATIONS

Flat   Low Convex   High Convex

EDGES

Entire   Irregular   Crenated

Fig. III.1. Elevations and edges of bacterial colonies.

genus *Corynebacterium.*

When growth occurs on artificial media *colonies* are formed. These can be described by elevation and by the type of edge the colony possesses (Fig. III.1).

When culturing the specimen the object of 'plating out' is to obtain single colonies from which pure cultures can be obtained should the infection be due to more than one species of microorganism. Techniques of plating out are well known, but it is imperative that the correct method is scrupulously followed to achieve single colonies on solid medium (see Fig. III.2). Where mixed bacterial populations can be expected, e.g. faeces, selective media are used to inhibit the growth of commensals, or un-

wanted bacteria.

Unless otherwise specified, incubation is usually at 37°C for 18–24 hours for media, broths, sugars, etc. A key to abbreviations used follows at the end of this introduction.

Anaerobic culture is best achieved in most routine laboratories by the use of the 'Gas-Pak'® System, Fig. III.3. This is a simple method and makes the dangerous use of hydrogen cylinders in the laboratory unnecessary. Growth on plates is visible through the clear plastic jar which need not therefore be taken down unnecessarily. A modification of the 'Gas-Pak'® System uses a carbon dioxide envelope in place of the hydrogen envelope when growth under CO_2 is required.

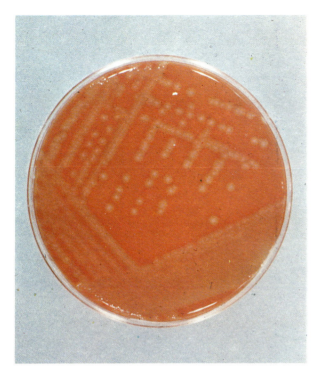

Fig. III.2. Techniques of plating out.
This figure shows a method of plating out
on solid medium to achieve isolated
single colonies and to make maximum
use of the media.

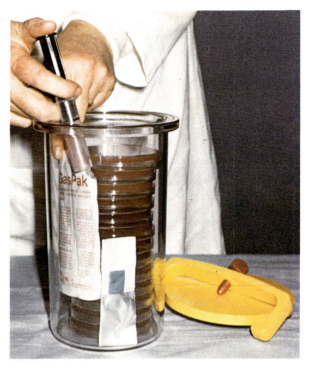

**Fig. III.3. The 'Gas-Pak'* jar and
envelope.*** 10 ml of water is injected
into the corner of the foil envelope which
is then placed upright in the jar. The
lid is then screwed down completely.
Note the anaerobic indicator.

Serological tests, where appropriate, are mentioned in the text.

Key to Abbreviations in Bacteriology Section

AR	Auramine-rhodamine stain
BA	Blood agar
BHI	Brain heart infusion broth
CA	Chocolate agar
CMM	Cooked meat medium
CSF	Cerebrospinal fluid
GA	Glucose agar
HBA	Horse blood agar
I/D	Intra-dermal
IM	Intra-muscular
IP	Intra-peritoneal
IV	Intravenous
LJ	Lowenstein Jensen medium
NA	Nutrient agar
RBC	Red blood cells
SA	Serum agar
SBA	Sheep blood agar
S/C	Subcutaneous
TCBS	Thiosulphate citrate bile-salts sucrose agar
TM	Thayer Martin medium
UTI	Urinary tract infection
XLD	Xylose lysine desoxycholate agar
ZN	Ziehl-Neelsen's stain

* Available from B.B.L., a division of Becton-Dickinson & Co.,
Cockeysville, Maryland 21030, U.S.A.

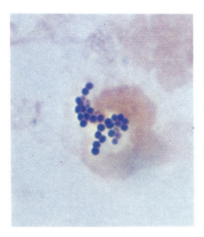

Fig. III.4. Gram stain of staphylococcal pus. The typical Gram positive cocci in 'grape-like' clusters is well shown. × 4308.

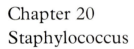

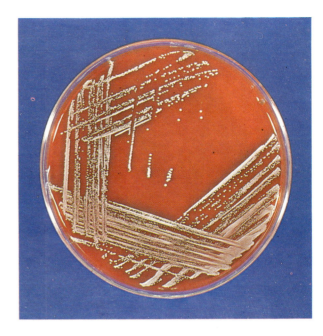

Fig. III.5. Colonial appearance of S. albus (epidermidis). Pure and profuse growth of the typical creamy-white colonies is shown here on BA after 18 hour incubation at 37°C.

Chapter 20
Staphylococcus

Staphylococci are Gram positive spherical cocci (or spheres) occurring typically in grape-like clusters, but sometimes in pairs. They may be irregular and their size varies from 0.8–1.0 μ. They are facultative anaerobes and biochemically active by fermentation. Coagulase positive staphylococci are designated *S. aureus* and this was meant to be an index of pathogenicity; it can no longer be considered so.

All members of the genus grow well on basal medium, and often possess a non-diffusable pigment which may be characteristic. They are all non-motile and non-sporing. In nature they are ubiquitous and are common commensals in man, especially in the nose and on the skin.

Fig. III.4 shows a Gram stain of staphylo-coccal pus illustrating the usual arrangement of staphylococci.

Cultural Characteristics

The convex colonies about 2–3 mm in diameter have an entire edge after incubation for 18–24 hours at 37°C. The pigment produced varies from white to lemon to golden yellow, dependent on the media used. Colonial pigment-forming ability lends easily to classification of the above colonies into *S. albus*, *S. citreus* and *S. aureus*, but is no index of pathogenicity. *S. albus* (*epidermidis*) is shown in Fig. III.5, and *S. aureus* in Fig. III.6. Pigmentation improves with time on the bench at room temperature as also does

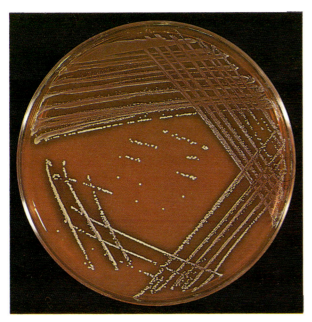

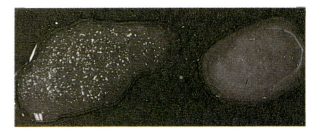

Fig. III.7. Slide coagulase test. On the one slide is shown a positive coagulase test, and on the right hand side is the negative control which shows no clumping.

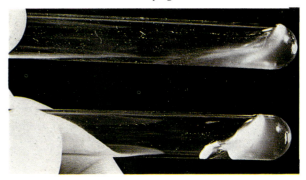

Fig. III.6. Colonial appearance of S. aureus. Note the golden-yellow appearance after careful plating out to single colonies following 18 hour incubation at 37 C on BA.

Fig. III.8. Tube coagulase test. Coagulation has occurred in the bottom tube indicating the organism is *S. aureus*. The top tube without coagulation is a negative control.

the size of the colonies. A particularly virulent type of *S. aureus* which is multi-antibiotic resistant presents a 'poached-egg' appearance.

Diagnosis

Selective media can be used, e.g. 8.5 per cent sodium chloride basal agar, or peptone broth with the same salt concentration. Differentiation of *S. aureus* is by the coagulase test. Coagulase is a soluble enzyme-like product of *S. aureus* which converts the fibrinogen of rabbit or human plasma into fibrin. There is a reasonably high correlation of pathogenicity and coagulase production which parallels DN Ase production.

The coagulase test can be performed two ways:

(a) *Bound coagulase* can be shown in about 30 seconds in a slide test, which is the method normally used. Undiluted plasma is added to a suspension of the test organism and the presence or absence of coagulation using a negative control is noted, see Fig. III.7.

(b) The less usual method demonstrates *soluble coagulase* by adding a few emulsified drops of the test culture to 1:10 sterile homologous human or rabbit plasma. The presence or absence in the tubes of coagulation after 2 hours in a water bath at 37°C compared with a negative control shows the reaction, see Fig. III.8.

If the result of the slide coagulase test is doubtful it should always be confirmed by the tube test, or better, by DNAse activity.

Fig. III.9. A typical phage plate.
Lysis, the cleared area on the confluent growth on the agar plate, shows the pattern which delineates the phage type of *S. aureus*.

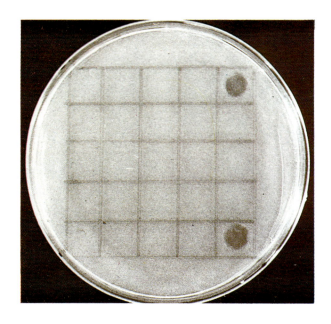

Table III.1. Classification of staphylococci by the coagulase test

Positive	Negative	Negative
S. aureus (pyogenes)	*S. albus (epidermidis)*	*S. citreus*
Golden yellow colonies	Creamy-white colonies	Lemon yellow colonies
↓	↓	↓
Pathogenic	May be pathogenic	Non-pathogenic

Staphylococci can be classified on the coagulase test and colonial morphology according to Table III.1.

Serology

Although available, serology is not routinely used. Three main serotypes with subtypes exist.

Phage Typing

Bacteriophages are perhaps best known in the case of *S. aureus* where their use is important in tracing outbreaks of epidemic sepsis. Bacteriophages lyse certain strains of *S. aureus* in particular patterns. Thus several hundred pat-terns may exist.

A standard WHO set of 24 different *S. aureus* bacteriophages are used at Routine Test Dilution (RTD) or 100 or 1000 × RTD. The organism under test is spread evenly over an agar plate which is pre-scored into 24 squares, it is allowed to dry at room temperature for 2–3 hours and one 0.01 ml drop of RTD of the respective phage is placed in each square. After incubation at 30°C for 18 hours the pattern of lysis which has occurred designates the particular phage type. Phage type 80/81 and close variants have been the cause of hospital-acquired infection over the past 15 years, see Fig. III.9.

Three major groups of phage types, are in general, responsible for their own type of infection.

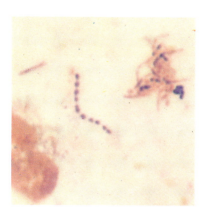

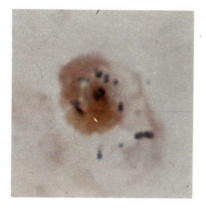

Fig. III.10. Gram stain of streptococcal pus. The classical picture of Gram positive cocci in chains is well shown in this photomicrograph. × 4308.

Fig. III.11. Gram stain of S. pneumoniae in sputum. The picture of the diplococcus presents no difficulty in diagnosis. Note that the organism is mainly intracellular. × 4308.

Chapter 21
Streptococcus

Streptococci are Gram positive spherical or ovoid cocci 0.5–1.0 μ in diameter occurring classically in chains, but in certain species in pairs, e.g. *S. pneumoniae*. They are catalase negative and usually non-motile, and all are non-sporing. Although they are facultatively anaerobic, some strains are strict anaerobes. Some are active biochemically and many strains possess a capsule. The genus usually requires enriched media for proper growth and can cause different types of haemolysis on various blood agar.

Fig. III.10 shows a Gram stain of *S. pyogenes* in classical chain formation.

Fig. III.11 is a photomicrograph of a Gram stain of sputum containing *S. pneumoniae*. This shows typical diplococci and it should be noted that the long axis of the organisms is horizontal.

Cultural Characteristics

Most members of this genus grow in colonies (1–2 mm in diameter) which are both opaque and very similar in shape and size. They are convex with an entire edge, and facultatively anaerobic.

Three different haemolytic reactions, designated α (partial), β (complete) and γ (none) occur on BA, are particularly well seen if the blood is sheep red cells. Haemolysis is apparent following 18–24 hour incubation at 37°C.

(a) α haemolytic streptococci are characterized by a greenish pigmentation surrounding the

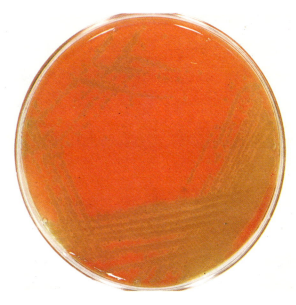

Fig. III.12. Typical alpha haemolytic streptococci on BA. Characteristic greenish or incomplete haemolysis of the blood around the small colony can be seen.

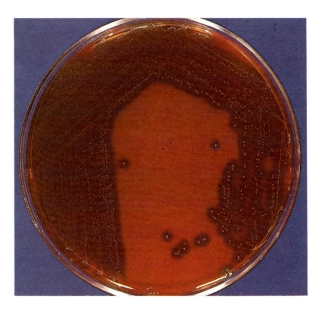

Fig. III.13. Beta haemolytic streptococci on BA. Characteristic clearing or complete haemolysis of the blood around the small colony can be seen.

colony with partial haemolysis of the blood in the agar, but no soluble haemolysin is produced, see Fig. III.12.

(b) β haemolytic streptococci give a clear zone of haemolysis of the blood in the agar, i.e. they possess a soluble haemolysin producing complete haemolysis of the blood adjacent to the colony. This zone of β haemolysis is much larger than that of α haemolysis and is so clear that one can easily see a finger through the medium. This haemolysis is shown in Fig. III.13, which is in marked contrast to α haemolysis.

(c) γ haemolytic streptococci produce neither haemolysin nor haemolysis. An example of this is *S. faecalis* shown in Fig. III.14. However, *S. faecalis* may also give α or β haemolysis.

Anaerobic streptococci show no haemolysis but are strictly anaerobic and are associated with a foul putrid odour. *Peptostreptococcus putridus* is the member most commonly found and is highly proteolytic.

Streptococcus viridans is not a class on its own, although determined by optochin resistance and bile insolubility. The group is pathogenic under certain circumstances and has been best described by Williams★ as containing five relevant taxa which he has called *salivarius*, *sanguis*, *milleri*, *mutans* and *mitior*, the latter in place of *mitis*.

★ Williams, R. E. O. (1973) Benefit and mischief from commensal bacteria. *J. Clin. Path.*, **26**, 811.

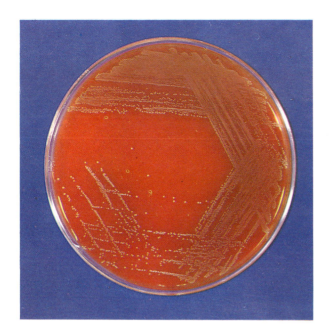

Fig. III.14. Gamma haemolytic streptococcus on BA. Note the absence of all haemolysis and the typical small opaque colonies of *S. faecalis* in the example shown here.

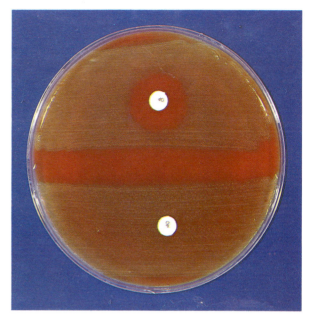

Fig. III.15. S. pneumoniae and the optochin test. A BA plate shows optochin sensitivity on the top half and resistance on the lower half. The top half is therefore *S. pneumoniae* and the lower *S. viridans* (see text). Note that both are α haemolytic.

In fact, it is beyond the scope of most busy routine laboratories to do more than report *S. viridans*. The quantitative assessment of specimens is the best guide to treatment.

S. pneumoniae apart from their characteristic appearance on Gram stain are proved by their sensitivity to an optochin disc and their bile solubility (see Fig. III.15). The serology of these types is discussed below.

S. faecalis (Enterococcus) is a common cause both of urinary tract infections and postoperative infections when the large bowel has been opened. It is a commensal in the bowel. *S. faecalis* grows on MacConkey agar as a small magenta coloured colony when compared say with *E. coli*. The difference in size is characteristic (see Fig. III.16).

The organism is notable for its salt resistance, it grows well in the presence of bile salts or on 6.5 per cent salt agar.

The Group D streptococci can be typed biochemically, but the majority are *S. faecalis*. They present large colonies on BA (2 mm diameter) and as is obvious from the above, they ferment lactose.

Diagnosis

Selective media can be used to inhibit staphylococci, e.g. horse or sheep blood agar containing 1/500,000 gentian violet. But SBA shows better haemolysis and thus aids diagnosis (Table III.2).

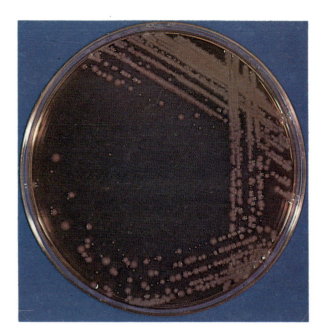

Fig. III.16. Mixture of S. faecalis and E. coli on MacConkey agar. The *S. faecalis* appears as a small lactose fermenting organism, compared with the much larger lactose fermenting colonies of the *E. coli*.

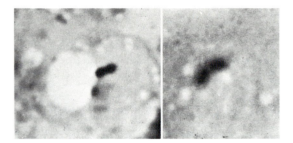

Fig. III.17. The Quellung reaction. The organism in both photos is *S. pneumoniae*. On the left hand side the organism is in the presence of *heterologous* antisera and methylene blue. There is no capsular swelling. On the right, the organism is present with *homologous* antisera and the capsular swelling is seen.

Serology

(a) *α haemolytic streptococci*: S. pneumoniae can be typed by the polysaccharide in the surrounding capsule and there are more than 75 serological types. Type 3 has the largest capsule and is the most virulent form. The capsular swelling (Quellung Reaction) is shown in Fig. III.17.

Somatic antigens are also used for differentiation, for example:
  (i) the cell wall antigen 'C substance' and
  (ii) the type specific 'M antigen' which is a protein independent of the type-specific capsular polysaccharide.

(b) *β haemolytic streptococci*: these can be subdivided into a number of broad groups determined by the chemical nature of the 'C-substance' or 'C-antigen'. This serves to divide the β haemolytic streptococci into the 18 Lancefield's Groups, A-T. (Note the absence of I or J.) See Table III.2.

Group A may be further subdivided by the Griffith's types which gives specific agglutination or a precipitin reaction using absorbed sera with the T and/or M or R protein. The M protein occurs in over 50 different serotypes.

Table III.2. Small opaque colonies 1 mm diameter on blood agar.

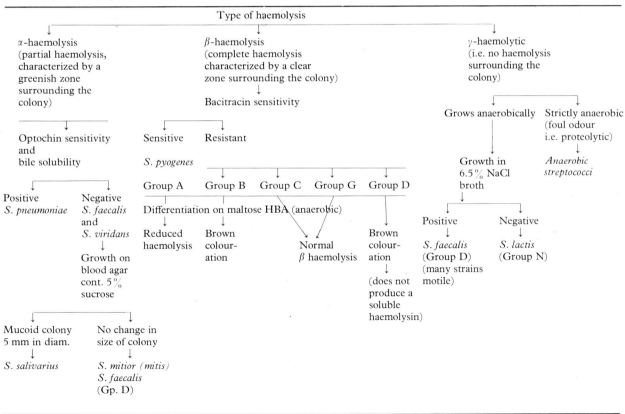

Chapter 22
Erysipelothrix

These microorganisms are considered to be members of the family *Corynebacteriaceae*. They are Gram positive, non-motile, non-sporing and catalase negative organisms. By fermentation they are biochemically active. They usually occur singly or in pairs and are $1-2 \times 0.3 \ \mu$ in size. They grow on enriched media and show α haemolysis on SBA.

E. rhusiopathiae (*E. insidiosa*) is the only pathogen of this genus.

In culture these organisms grow to small α haemolytic colonies on SBA.

Diagnosis

The organism is difficult to culture from swabs alone, but a biopsy specimen, after homogenization, cultured for 48 hours in 1 per cent glucose broth can then be subcultured onto SBA and is usually diagnostic.

Chapter 23
Listeria

Listeria monocytogenes is important as an unusual cause of meningitis. These organisms are considered to be members of the *Corynebacteriaceae* family. In young cultures they are non-sporing Gram positive bacilli, generally curved (cf. Corynebacteria, Chapter 24) and $2–3 \times 0.5$ μ in size. They are often seen in pairs because of the method of cell division, and they are motile, catalase positive, aerobic and biochemically active by fermentation. On sheep blood agar (SBA) β haemolysis is the rule. *Listeria* are capable of growth at $4°C$. The only pathogenic member of the genus is *L. monocytogenes*.

Diagnosis

Growth occurs on SBA or 0.5 per cent glucose agar (GA) under 8–10 per cent CO_2. There is typical *tumbling motility* after 6 hours at $25°C$ in brain heart infusion broth (BHI). It should be noted that after incubation at $37°C$ these microorganisms are only feebly motile. Colonies are small and β haemolytic (often mistaken for *S. pyogenes*). For this reason a representative selection of the colonies should be Gram stained.

Diagnosis can also be established by demonstrating a rise in the agglutination titre.

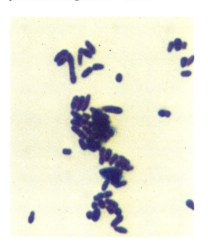

Chapter 24
Corynebacterium

Classification

This genus is divided into four major serological types on the basis of somatic ('O') and flagella ('H') antigens. These are designated as types 1–4. Types 1, 4a and 4b are the common serotypes producing disease in man.

Corynebacteria are irregularly staining Gram positive bacilli, sometimes with volutin or meta-chromatic granules giving a club-shaped appearance. This is because of the way they divide— snapping and bending abruptly—leading to pallisade formation or the more classical 'Chinese letter' configuration. In size they are $0.3 \times 3\ \mu$, but they are often pleomorphic.

The *Corynebacteria* are non-motile, and they do not possess a capsule. They are non-sporing but are facultatively anaerobic. The catalase reaction is positive and they are usually bio-chemically active. Some species produce pigment and some exotoxins. Fig. III.18 shows the typical pallisade arrangement of the *Coryne-bacteria*.

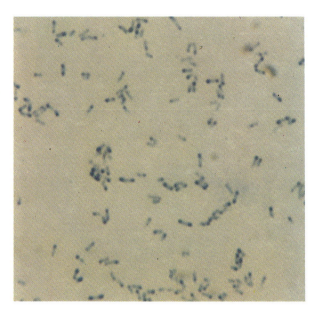

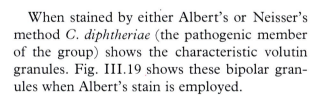

Fig. III.19. C. diphtheriae stained by Albert's method. The bipolar granules are readily visible and are diagnostic when taken in conjunction with the pallisade or 'Chinese Letter' formation shown in Fig. III.18. × 4342.

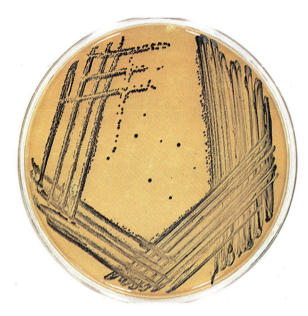

Fig. III.20. C. diphtheriae var gravis on blood tellurite agar. Note the crenated edge, and black colony and the absence of haemolysis.

When stained by either Albert's or Neisser's method *C. diphtheriae* (the pathogenic member of the group) shows the characteristic volutin granules. Fig. III.19 shows these bipolar granules when Albert's stain is employed.

Cultural Characteristics

These organisms grow best at 37°C on BA or serum agar (SA). They present as greyish colonies 1–2 mm in size. Their edge is normally entire, but may be crenated.

On selective enriched media, such as potassium tellurite, colonies are much smaller even after 48 hours incubation but *C. diphtheriae* biotypes grow on this medium with a characteris-

tic morphology. The colonies are black, ranging from 1–5 mm in size—all other species are grey in colour. Fig. III.20 shows *C. diphtheriae var gravis* growing on potassium tellurite blood agar.

Table III.3. Colonial morphology on tellurite blood agar after 2–3 days at 35°C

C. diphtheriae var gravis	The colony is 3–5 mm in diameter, flat with a black raised centre, and a crenated edge. The colony has radial striations and can be described as a 'daisy-head'.
C. diphtheria var mitis	The colony is 2–4 mm in diameter, black in colour with a 'poached egg' appearance, i.e. central elevation. It is darker than *C. diphtheriae var gravis*, and has an entire edge.
C. diphtheriae var intermedius	Small colony approximately 1 mm in size, and resembles a miniature *gravis* type.

Table III.4. Biochemical tests of Corynebacteria

	Glucose	Sucrose	Starch
C. equi	−	−	−
C. hofmannii	−	−	−
C. diphtheriae var gravis	+(+acid)	−	+(+acid)
C. diphtheria var mitis	+(+acid)	−	−
C. diphtheriae var intermedius	+(+acid)	−	−
C. xerosis	+(+acid)	+	−

Diagnosis

The selective tellurite agar allows of differentiation from the size, shape and colonial appearance of colonies due to *C. diphtheriae*.

Table III.3 details the characteristic colonial morphology after 48 hours on blood tellurite agar.

Further identification can be achieved by fermentation tests as follows in Table III.4.

Serology

The three biotypes of *C. diphtheriae* can also be further subdivided by either serology or phage typing.

Virulence (or Toxigenicity)

Not all strains of *C. diphtheriae* are virulent, but this can be measured by the Römer test, in which a guinea pig partially protected by antitoxin shows local necrosis after intradermal injection of a toxin-producing organism. A fully protected control pig must be used. Toxigenicity can also be demonstrated by the use of an agar-gel diffusion test.

Chapter 25
Mycobacteria

DEFINITION

The mycobacteria are non-motile slender beaded Gram positive bacilli which stain poorly by Gram's method. Typically they are 'acid-fast' due to the waxy material in their cell walls. Non-sporing and aerobic they require enriched media for growth. Colonies are often pigmented, catalase positive and biochemically active by oxidation. Some species are pathogenic for man, others are saprophytic.

They are ubiquitous in nature. The pathogenic species are the mammalian tubercle bacilli, viz. *Mycobacterium tuberculosis* (the human type of tubercle bacillus), the main host of which is man, and *M. bovis* (the bovine type of tubercle bacillus), which is pathogenic both to man and

also to cattle, which is the main host although other animals are affected.

Another group which are acid-fast, and are not tubercle bacilli yet are associated with human disease have been named the 'atypical' or 'anonymous' mycobacteria. These have been divided into four further groups (Runyon).

A further group cause chronic skin ulcers—these are *M. ulcerans* and *M. marinum* (*balnei*).

The fourth and final group is *M. leprae* the causative agent of leprosy.

Mycobacterium tuberculosis

M. tuberculosis is the cause of human tuberculosis. They are poorly staining Gram positive

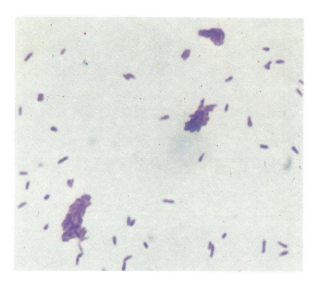

Fig. III.21. Tight cording effect of M. tuberculosis when stained by Ziehl-Neelsen stain. Typical cording effect of the acid-fast bacilli can be seen in several places. × 4342.

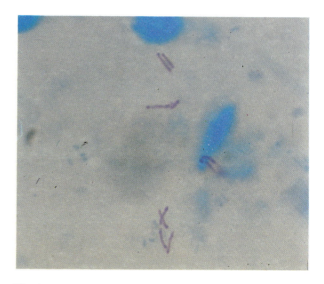

Fig. III.22. Acid-fast bacilli in the sputum of a patient with pulmonary tuberculosis. Note the slender slightly curved acid-fast organisms, against the blue background of leucocytes. × 4342.

bacilli, which may be slightly curved, but are slender. Variable in size, they are approximately $3 \mu \times 0.3 \mu$ and are acid-alcohol fast.

Fig. III.21 shows the typical tight cording effect when stained by ZN from a culture on Lowenstein-Jensen egg media.

Fig. III.22 shows the typical red acid-fast staining rods with a blue background of a sputum specimen from a patient with pulmonary tuberculosis.

CULTURAL CHARACTERISTICS

M. tuberculosis does not grow on basal media. Primary culture is performed on enriched media —the usual one being LJ egg media which is incubated at 37°C aerobically. Growth is slow but may be visible after 14 days at the earliest, but 6–8 weeks incubation or even 12 weeks may be required for growth (see Fig. III.23).

The colonies appear as a rough, dry, pigmented, irregular type of colony, which is difficult to emulsify, and is creamy-white in colour, later turning to buff.

DIAGNOSIS

M. tuberculosis is not a commensal, and the demonstration of the typical acid-alcohol-fast cording bacilli cultured from a specimen is presumptive evidence of infection.

Further identification is performed by using

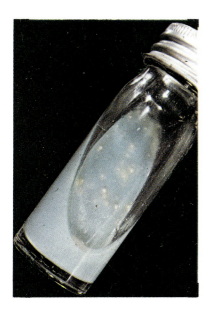

Fig. III.23. M. tuberculosis on a Lowenstein-Jensen slope after 6 weeks incubation at 37°C. Pale yellow, rough colonies on the green LJ slope can be seen.

the niacin test and pathogenicity in the guinea pig. If both of these are positive the organism is *M. tuberculosis*.

SEROLOGY

No tests are available in the laboratory.

ANIMAL PATHOGENICITY

The guinea pig is the most susceptible laboratory animal to both human and bovine *M. tuberculosis*.

The specimen to be inoculated is injected S/C into the hind leg of the animal (usually 2 animals are used). One animal is sacrificed after 6 weeks when a characteristic picture may be seen; there may be necrotic ulceration at the site of inoculation, and there is involvement of the inguinal and para-aortic lymph glands, which are either enlarged or show chronic lesions. The spleen and later the liver may then become involved. The lymph nodes, liver, spleen, etc. are then sectioned for the presence of acid-fast bacilli, thus fulfilling Koch's postulates. The second guinea pig is sacrificed at 12 weeks if the previous animal was negative.

Atypical or Anonymous Mycobacteria

These have been divided into four groups (Runyon) depending on the capacity of the cultures to become pigmented on exposure to light.

Mycobacteria 67

GROUP I. PHOTOCHROMOGENS

These become yellow on exposure to light, i.e. they do not produce pigment in the dark. They are non-pathogenic for the guinea pig. The most important pathogen in this group is *Mycobacterium kansasii* which may cause a human pulmonary infection which is indistinguishable from *M. tuberculosis*. It is niacin negative, and does not produce tight cording and takes more than 5 days to grow.

GROUP II. SCOTOCHROMOGENS

These are widely distributed in nature. They produce orange colonies in the darkness of the incubator. They are non-pathogenic for guinea pigs, and also are niacin negative. One species, *M. scrofulaceum*, may cause cervical adenitis in children. This does not produce tight cording and takes more than 5 days to grow.

GROUP III. NON-CHROMOGENS

These organisms produce no pigment in the dark or light, they include *M. intracellulare* (formerly called Battey strain), which is so closely related to *M. avium* that some authorities regard them as members of the same species in cases of pulmonary tuberculosis not due to *M. tuberculosis*. They do not produce tight cording, take more than 5 days to grow and are niacin resistant. *M. avium* is the cause of rural rather than urban infection in man (grows at 45°C), as also does *M. zenopi*. It is niacin negative, and non-pathogenic for the guinea pig.

GROUP IV. RAPID GROWERS

These are usually saphophytes or commensals, so may lead to false diagnosis of UTI, etc; they take less than 5 days to grow. But see also: Runyon, E. H. (1974) Ten Mycobacterial Pathogens, *Tubercle*, **55**, 235.

Mycobacterium ulcerans

DEFINITION

This is an acid fast organism which grows at an optimum temperature of 32°C. It is strictly a human pathogen, but does not appear to spread from man to man. The organism seems to enter the skin by some form of abrasion, usually on the leg or arm.

DIAGNOSIS

Smears or better, biopsy from the edge of the lesion show strongly acid-alcohol-fast organisms. Growth at 32°C occurs after 6–8 weeks. The bacilli are arranged in cords and are niacin negative.

ANIMAL PATHOGENICITY

Not pathogenic for guinea pigs, but ulceration occurs when injected into the foot pad of the mouse.

Table III.5. Differentiation between *M. ulcerans* and *M. marinum.*

	M. ulcerans	*M. marinum*
Climate	Temperate	Temperate
Type of Ulcer	Progressive	Rapid and self limiting
Temp. of Growth	30°–33°C (Poorly) (not at 37°C)	30°–33°C (but also 37°C)
Mouse inoculation	Oedema and ulceration	Oedema and pus
Tissues	Invasive	Scanty effect
Pigmentation	Nil	Yellow when exposed to light.

Backyard swimming pools are a not uncommon source of *M. marinum.*

Mycobacterium marinum (balnei)

DEFINITION

Acid-fast bacilli which are long, and banded, rather larger than the human tubercle bacilli. Grows only between 30° and 32°C, after two weeks incubation (grow poorly at 37°C). After exposure to light they may become bright golden in colour.

DIAGNOSIS

Acid-fast bacilli detected from granulomatous skin lesions, they are niacin negative.

ANIMAL PATHOGENICITY

No effect in guinea pigs, but I/D injection into the foot pad of the mouse is followed after a few days of inflammation, by slowly advancing oedema and ulceration.

Mycobacterium leprae

DEFINITION

M. leprae is a straight or slightly slender bacillus, with pointed, rounded or club-shaped ends. Acid-fast, but not alcohol-fast, it requires 5 per cent sulphuric acid for decolourization. It is Gram positive, and cannot be cultured on arti-

Fig. III.25. Nocardia species. Modified Ziehl-Neelsen stain of pus from a patient with nocardia showing the typical acid-fast branching filaments. × 4342.

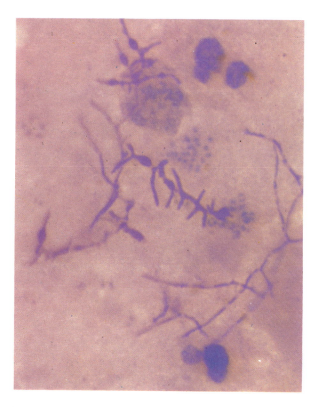

Fig. III.24. M. leprae in tissue. × 2525.

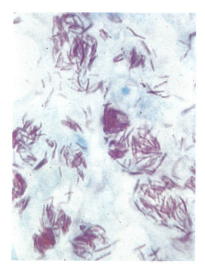

ficial media. It is the causative organism of leprosy. Fig. III.24 shows the organism in such a lesion.

DIAGNOSIS

This is by detection of acid-fast bacilli from impression smears, or lymph exudates, or from scrapings of the nasal mucosa, using 5 per cent sulphuric acid instead of the conventional 25 per cent sulphuric acid as normally used in Ziehl-Neelsen stain.

Chapter 26
Nocardia

Nocardiosis is caused by *Nocardia asteroides* and *N. brasiliensis*. They are partially acid-fast and may be mistaken for *M. tuberculosis* in sputum and other exudates. Nocardiosis can present as a pneumonia, lung or brain abscess or as a bacter-aemia. The disease may be acute or chronic, but in every instance is severe and life-threatening.

Unlike the anaerobic actinomyces, *N. aster-oides* has frequently been found in soil. *N. brasiliensis* has not been so isolated, but is a cause of mycetomata.

Granules are not formed by *Nocardia*; the organism appears as Gram positive or weakly acid-fast delicate branching systems in specimens (Fig. III.25).

All the specimens may be cultured on ordinary

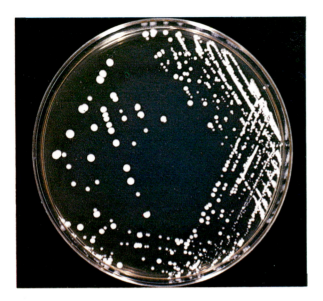

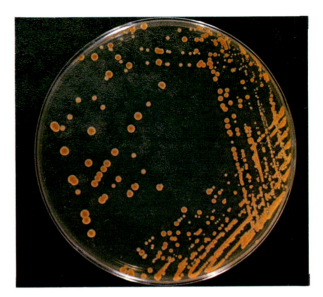

Fig. III.26. Nocardia species. Upper surface of *N. asteroides* grown on basal agar at 37°C for 7 days showing the typical white granular colonies which are 1 mm in diameter and tend to dig into the surface of the agar.

Fig. III.27 (top right). Nocardia species. Under surface of *N. asteroides* showing the typical yellow colour of the colonies.

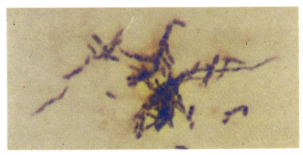

Fig. III.28. Nocardia species. Gram stain of a culture of *N. asteroides* showing poorly staining Gram positive branching, filamentous bacilli. × 4342.

media at 37°C. *N. asteroides* is granular, glabrous or irregularly folded, the colour varying from white to yellow to deep orange (Figs. III.26, 27).

Pigmentation and the amount of aerial mycelium vary considerably. The colonies adhere firmly to the underlying medium. The size of the colony however, is only 2–3 mm, similar to a staphylococcal colony.

The colonies stain poorly by Gram's method, but appear as Gram positive branching bacilli (Fig. III.28). When stained by modified Ziehl-Neelsen stain they are weakly acid-fast and also have the typical branching filaments (Fig. III.29).

N. asteroides shows no growth in 0.4 per cent gelatin after two weeks at 37°C whereas *N. brasiliensis* grows well.

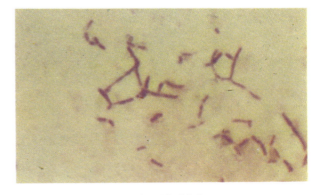

Fig. III.29. Nocardia species. Modified Ziehl-Neelsen stain of a culture of *N. asteroides* showing the typical acid-fast branching bacilli. × 4342.

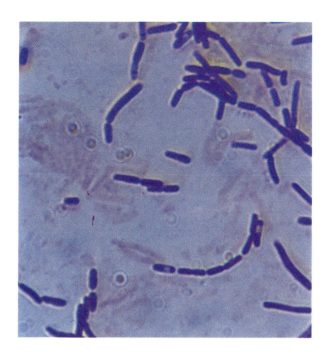

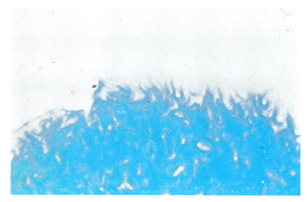

Fig. III.30. B. cereus stained by Gram. Gram positive bacilli in chains, note that some organisms are producing spores. × 4342.

Fig. III.31. Medusa head appearance of B. anthracis. This is well shown on a low power view. × 334.

III.31

Chapter 27
Bacillus

Bacillus anthracis and *B. cereus* are the only pathogenic members of this group. The former causes anthrax and the latter food poisoning. Of course, like all other microorganisms, in the severely compromised host, e.g. a renal transplant patient who is heavily immunosuppressed, any organism may cause disease.

In young cultures bacilli are 4–9 × 1.5 μ in size, often in chains, they form spores and are moderately heat resistant. In contrast to other non-pathogenic members of the genus, *B. anthracis* is non-motile, but *B. cereus* is usually motile. Both are catalase positive and some possess capsules. They grow well on basal agar, are facultatively anaerobic and are also biochemically active by fermentation. Fig. III.30 shows the organism in chains with typical spore formation.

Cultural Characteristics

On basal agar colonies best show their morphology at 28°C where they are about 3 mm in size. *B. anthracis* typically has a 'medusa head' appearance (see Fig. III.31). Little, if any, haemolysis occurs on BA.

Diagnosis

Diagnosis is usually made on cultural characteristics, motility, capsular staining and the classical 'inverted fir tree' effect in gelatin medium.

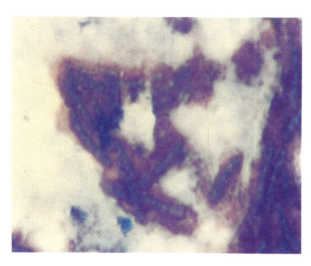

Fig. III.32. McFadyean's reaction with B. anthracis. Blood film stained by polychrome methylene blue shows bacilli staining blue surrounded by a reddish granular material, which is the broken-down capsule. × 4342.

Confirmation of the diagnosis is by injection of the organism into a guinea pig and observation of the characteristic post-mortem findings. Death normally occurs within 4 days of inoculation. Smears taken from heart blood and the spleen are stained with polychrome methylene blue; in these, the bacilli are blue and are surrounded by a purplish-red granular staining effect (McFadyean's Reaction) which is the disrupted capsular material. This effect is noted only with *B. anthracis* (see Fig. III.32).

Serology

Confirmation is obtained by the Ascoli precipitin test which utilizes as the antigen a post-mortem tissue extract which is boiled in saline. The antigen is then layered on anthrax antiserum and a ring is formed at the junction.

The capsular polypeptide is composed of D-glutamic acid and is the basis of serology of virulent strains.

Chapter 28
Clostridium

The pathogenic members of the species are *Clostridium tetani*, *C. welchii (perfringens)*, *oedematiens*, *septicum* and *botulinum*. Most other members are soil and dust saprophytes or commensals especially of the alimentary tract of animals and man where a few species may be pathogenic causing severe gastroenteritis occasionally. For example 'pig-bel' in New Guinea natives is caused by a strain of *C. welchii*, type C.

In young cultures the organisms are Gram positive with spores which normally distend them. Except for *C. welchii* most members are motile, are non-acid-fast, catalase negative and grow well on basal agar under anaerobic conditions. Some members are facultatively anaerobic, others, e.g. *C. tetani* are strict anaerobes. Some are biochemically active by fermentation.

Some species produce powerful exotoxins, some are saccharolytic whilst others are offensively proteolytic.

Clostridium welchii (perfringens)

This is the organism most often responsible for clinical gas gangrene. It is a large Gram positive bacillus about $4–6 \times 1\ \mu$ in size generally with squarish ends, although these may be rounded, and the most virulent form is a somewhat shorter rod with definite square ends. The organism usually appears singly. When isolated from a fresh infection it possesses a characteristic capsule the shape of which is of considerable help

Fig. III.33. Clostridium welchii (perfringens) on Gram stain. Note the characteristic square ends to the rod. × 4342.

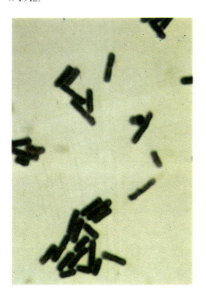

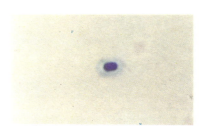

Fig. III.34. C. welchii (perfringens) capsular stain (Muir's). Note the organism is pinkish and the capsule colourless to blue. The size and fragmentation of the capsule taken in conjunction with the intactness of the leucocytes is an indication of virulence. × 4342.

Fig. III.35. 'Stormy clot' in litmus milk with C. welchii (perfringens). A provisional diagnosis of gas gangrene is made on Gram and Muir's stains and in a matter of 5–6 hours this can be confirmed by the litmus milk reaction. The extensive gas and acid production can be seen in the tube on the left, compared with the control on the right. This can influence the surgeon's treatment, e.g. by blood transfusion, antisera etc.

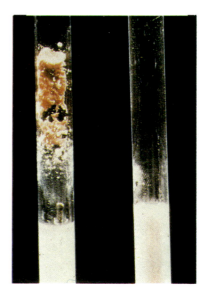

in determining the progress and likely outcome of the disease. It may have oval sub-terminal spores and is non-motile, saccharolytic and slightly proteolytic. Although an anaerobe, it is micro-aerophilic but grows rapidly in anaerobic culture.

The typical morphology of *C. welchii* stained with Gram is shown in Fig. III.33. An organism stained with Muir's capsular stain is illustrated in Fig. III.34. As the result of Muir's capsular stain constitutes a medical emergency not only from the diagnostic point of view but also from that of prognosis, the method is included.

CULTURAL CHARACTERISTICS

On horse blood agar (HBA) after anaerobic culture in a Gas Pak® System at 37°C for 18–24 hours the organism appears as greyish to colourless colonies 2–3 mm in diameter. Colonies are usually surrounded by a zone of complete haemolysis and sometimes by a secondary ring of incomplete haemolysis.

The organism ferments most sugars with much gas production. In litmus milk there is rapid (6 hour) fermentation of lactose and this saccharolytic activity causes disruption of the clot by acid forming the diagnostic 'stormy clot' (see Fig. III.35).

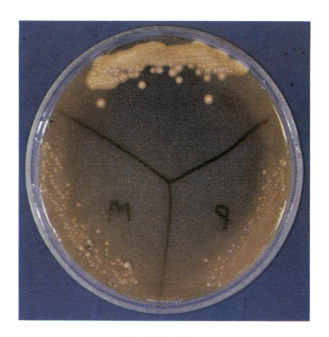

Fig. III.36. Neomycin-Nägler plate with antitoxin for the identification of C. welchii (perfringens). Note the precipitation of the lecithin in the control third of the plate compared with the lack of precipitation, by the neutralization of the toxins on the other two segments of the plate (labelled P. & M. for polyvalent and monovalent antitoxin).

DIAGNOSIS

Selective media in the form of neomycin Nägler plates (Willis and Hobbs medium) are used. Neomycin is added (200 μg/ml) to stop the growth of other bacteria, and the *C. welchii* growth produces lecithinase which precipitates the lecithin from the egg yolk in the medium. This occurs around the colony and spreads widely.

Further identification is by the use of mono- and polyvalent gas gangrene antisera spread over one third of the surface of the above plate. One third acts as a control (no antitoxin), another one third has polyvalent antisera (*C. welchii*, *septicum* and *oedematiens*) and the final third has monovalent *C. welchii* antitoxin spread on it.

Where the toxin produced by the organism is neutralized by the antisera *no* precipitation of lecithin occurs, thus there is no opalescence around these colonies when compared with the control area (see Fig. III.36). Growth in Robertson's cooked meat medium is typically saccharolytic.

The diagnosis of food poisoning due to *C. welchii* can be made from an actual count of the number of organisms per gram of faeces. The normal stool has less than 10^3 organisms per gram, whereas the stools of patients with food poisoning usually contain more than 10^6 organisms per gram (90 per cent of cases).

Serology

Five serological types (A–E) can be distinguished according to the exotoxins produced. Type A is most commonly associated with gas gangrene—this produces an alpha toxin, further, a subgroup within Type A is frequently associated with *C. welchii* food poisoning. Types B–E are normally seen in animal diseases.

Animal Pathogenicity

Virulence varies, but some strains are extremely pathogenic for guinea pigs after S/C or I.M. injection of an inoculum from Robertson's CMM. A control animal is normally protected by prior injection of 300–500 u of *C. welchii* antitoxin. Death can occur in the unprotected animal in as short a time as 12 hours with characteristic post-mortem changes. The protected pig remains alive and well.

This test of animal pathogenicity is enhanced by the addition of calcium ions in the form of 5 per cent calcium chloride with the inoculum.

Method of Performing Muir's Capsular Stain

There is no satisfactory method of staining capsules but they may be detected by simple methods (e.g. Gram stain). If these fail, then more complex procedures such as Muir's stain can be tried.

The smear is prepared in the usual manner and dried in air without fixation.

Make up A.M.T. Mordant before staining.

1 Strong carbol fuchsin (steaming) $\frac{1}{2}$–1 min
2 Wash with alcohol.   5–10 sec
3 Wash in running water.   2–3 min
4 A.M.T. mordant.   30 sec
5 Wash alternately in running water and alcohol until pale red.
6 Wash with water.
7 Loeffler's methylene blue $\frac{1}{2}$–1 min
8 Tip off and blot dry.

RESULT

Correctly   Organisms—red
              Capsules—blue (but may be different shades of blue).

A.M.T. MORDANT

Aluminium potash (sat. aqueous solution)	10 ml
Mercuric chloride (sat. aqueous solution)	4 ml
Tannic acid (20 per cent aqueous solution)	4 ml
Chloroform	few drops

Mix freshly before use.

Clostridium septicum

These are Gram positive bacilli varying greatly in size from 4–6 × 0.6 μ, but shapes may be very different. Oval sporing forms usually occur and distend the organism. The spores are usually central or subterminal. Older cultures may appear Gram negative on staining. They are neither motile nor encapsulated, nor do they have saccharolytic activity. They are ubiquitous in origin but still produce a powerful exotoxin.

CULTURAL CHARACTERISTICS

These *Clostridia* are strictly anaerobic with colonies 3–4 mm in size after 48 hours incubation at 37°C. Haemolysis surrounds the colonies and has a tendency to spread. Most members ferment sugars.

SEROLOGY

Considerable cross-antigenicity exists between *C. septicum*, *C. oedematiens* (v.i.) and *C. chauvoei*. *C. septicum* possesses two somatic antigens (1 and 2) and five 'H' antigens (a–e) giving in all a combination of six groups. Exotoxins are produced by alpha, beta, gamma and delta (α, β, γ, δ) strains.

ANIMAL PATHOGENICITY

IM injection of the organism produces an inflammatory reaction with little gas formation in the tissues.

Clostridium oedematiens (C. novyi)

In many ways this resembles *C. welchii*, but the organism is larger, more pleomorphic and a much stricter anaerobe. In itself it is rapidly inactivated by air (see Chapter 17) and its motility is similarly impaired. Although saccharolytic, no capsule is produced. Spores are oval, central or subterminal. The organism is ubiquitous in nature but produces an exotoxin.

CULTURAL CHARACTERISTICS

Spreading growth is very characteristic on BA and most strains produce a degree of haemolysis around the colony. Certain strains ferment sugars.

SEROLOGY

C. oedematiens includes four main types (A–D) dependent upon their toxin production. Type A is an occasional cause of gas gangrene in man. Other types cause infections in animals.

Clostridium tetani

This organism causes tetanus in humans and animals, and it is ubiquitous in nature, e.g. soil, dust, rose thorns, etc. In a Gram stain it presents as a straight slender positive rod (2.5–0.5 μ) with rounded ends. It usually shows a distended terminal 'drum-stick' spore but the organism is non-motile. In ageing cultures the organism tends to become Gram negative. The

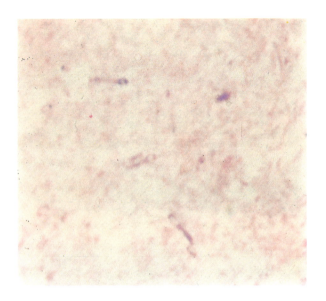

Fig. III.37. A typical example of C. tetani on Gram stain. The subterminal or 'drum-stick' spore of *C. tetani* is easily seen. × 4342.

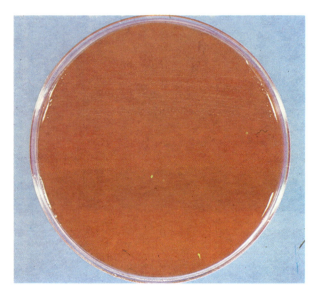

Fig. III.38. Swarming culture of C. tetani. The BA plate has been plated out with a culture of *C. tetani*. Note that the organism has swarmed from the site of the inoculation.

organism is weakly proteolytic but the spores are highly resistant both to heat and desiccation. Being a strict anaerobe this condition of culture is obligatory (see Fig. III.37).

CULTURAL CHARACTERISTICS

The organism is a strict anaerobe and can easily be killed by oxygen. It grows on most media, but best on an enriched medium where the colonies are rough and tend to swarm over the surface of the agar (see Fig. III.38). It is killed within a wide temperature range, and is not biochemically active.

SEROLOGY

Ten serological types can be distinguished from flagellar antigens. Type VI consists of non-flagellate strains, but all strains produce the same neurotoxin; non-toxigenic strains may belong to the same group.

The exotoxin, which is the most important clinically, varies from strain to strain and is also dependent on the media used. Tetanus toxin is extremely powerful, second only in effect to that produced by *C. botulinum*.

ANIMAL PATHOGENICITY

Two mice are used, one protected by 750 units of tetanus antitoxin prior to inoculation. Both

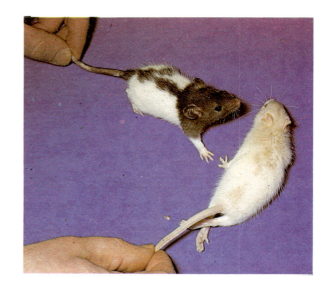

Fig. III.39. Animal inoculation of C. tetani. Note that the mouse on the left shows no disability, whereas the mouse on the right, twitches his tail and leg towards the site of injection.

mice are then injected S/C into the vein at the base of the tail with a culture of the test organism. The unprotected mouse dies within 48 hours with typical signs of tetanus starting with 'local tetanus', i.e. twitching of the tail towards the side of injection (see Fig. III.39). The protected mouse shows no disability.

Clostridium botulinum

C. botulinum is the causative agent of botulism in man. Although a rare disease, the organism is ubiquitous in nature. It is a short anaerobic Gram positive bacillus measuring 5×1 μ. It is motile, and spores are oval and subterminal and the organism is not capsulated. Optimal growth temperature is 35°C. On staining, the organism is Gram variable particularly in older cultures.

CULTURAL CHARACTERISTICS

Colonies are irregularly round with a fimbriated edge, but show much variation. They are translucent and 3 mm in diameter. Although biochemically active, the different serotypes vary both in saccharolytic and proteolytic activity.

SEROLOGY

Six main serotypes, A–F, have been shown on the basis of their distinct antigenic toxins. Types A, B and E are those most frequently associated

Chapter 29
Actinomyces

with botulism in man, although Types C, D and F have sometimes been incriminated. The exotoxin is destroyed when exposed to a temperature of 50°C for 40 min. Type A toxin has been isolated as a pure protein and is probably the most toxic substance known to man.

ANIMAL PATHOGENICITY

A similar test to that used with *C. tetani* is available, protecting only one animal of the two inoculated. The injection of *C. botulinum* is IP.

This genus of micro-aerophilic to anaerobic obligate parasites is possibly more closely related to the bacteria than to the higher fungi.

The anaerobic *Actinomyces israelii* normally inhabits the mouth and is often found in association with carious teeth and in tonsillar crypts. It is not an inhabitant of natural substrates. There is also a non-pathogenic facultative anaerobe *A. naeslundii* found in the normal mouth and saliva. A third member, *A. propionicus* has been isolated from lacrimal canaliculitis, and a fourth, *A. eriksonii* has been isolated from lung abscesses and pleural fluid in a few patients. *A. bovis* causes 'lumpy jaw' in cattle but can be pathogenic for man.

Actinomycosis is a chronic suppurative disease

Fig. III.40. Actinomyces species.
Gram stain of a 'sulphur granule' which
has been crushed between two slides.
This shows a central Gram positive
filamentous mass, surrounded by
Gram negative radiating clubs hence the
term 'ray fungus'. × 1336.

Fig. III.41. Actinomyces species.
Gram stain of pus from a patient with
actinomycosis which shows irregularly
staining Gram positive, branching
filaments amongst the pus debris.
× 4342.

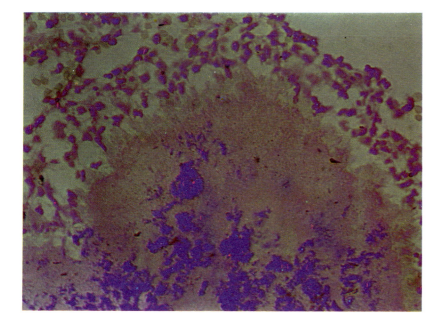

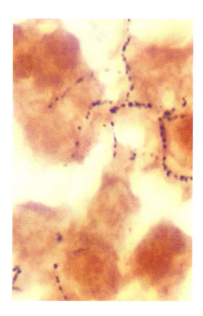

characterized by peripheral spread to contiguous
tissues without limitation by anatomical barriers.
Sinus formation commonly occurs in the neck,
then the abdomen and finally the thorax. These
drain a discharge containing yellow colonies 1–2
mm in size called 'sulphur granules'. Infection
is endogenous and is not transmitted from man
to man.

The presence of other bacteria in actinomycotic lesions suggests they may be a necessary part
of the disease. The most common 'associates', as
these other bacteria are called, are similar to
Haemophilus, fusiforms, anaerobic streptococci
or other Gram negative bacteria. For precise
identification of the *Actinomyces* rigid exclusion
of these 'associates' is necessary.

Laboratory diagnosis is often suggested by
taking the granules caught in a web dressing
or in aspirated pus. These should be mounted
on a slide, crushed and then Gram stained. Here,
Actinomyces appear as Gram positive filaments,
branching, often beaded or club-shaped, sometimes with diphtheroid-like elements. The typical granule shows peripheral clubs, hence the
name, 'ray fungus' (Fig. III.40). Branching,
beaded, Gram positive filaments are seen under
oil immersion (Fig. III.41). The main laboratory
finding is the presence of Gram positive filaments or bacteria which neither grow aerobically,
nor on Sabouraud's medium. There is no animal
toxicity.

Cultures are made anaerobically on BA and

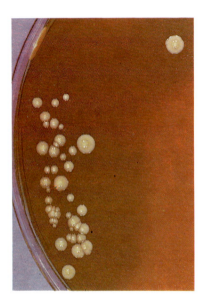

Fig. III.42. Actinomyces species.
A. israelii colonies after 48 hours.

examined every 2–3 days. At 24–48 hours *A. israelii* colonies appear as a loose spidery mycelial growth (Fig. III.42). At 7–10 days it presents characteristically as raised and rough colonies with a 'molar tooth' shape.

A. bovis, and *A. naeslundii*, *A. propionicus* and *A. eriksonii* all present different colonies on BHI agar from *A. israelii*. The first three are smooth and round but *A. eriksonii* present flat, granular colonies with a dense 'hyphal' cone. Biochemical reactions determine the precise nature of the *Actinomyces*.

Chapter 30
Haemophilus

Haemophilus are Gram negative, pleomorphic bacilli, which are non-motile, facultatively anaerobic, encapsulated and do not grow on basal agar, unless supplied with two factors, X (haematin), and/or V (co-enzyme 1).

They are Gram negative cocco-bacilli 1.5 μ × 0.5 μ in size.

Cultural Characteristics

Growth on chocolate agar after 24 hours incubation at 37°C appears as small greyish colonies 2 mm in diameter; if both X and V factors are provided and required, satellitism can be demonstrated (see Fig. III.43).

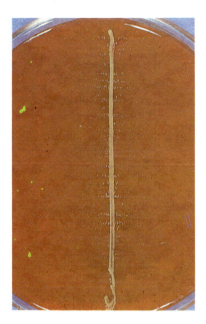

Fig. III.43. Satellitism of H. influenzae. The *H. influenzae* has been plated out over the entire surface of a BA plate, then *S. aureus* has been streaked down the centre. The haematin in the blood provides X factor, while the staphylococcus supplies the V factor, thus small colonies can be seen close to the staphylococcus, but are absent from the rest of the BA.

Diagnosis

Diagnosis is based on the X and V factor requirements, and six species are regarded as pathogenic:

(i) *H. ducreyi*
(ii) *H. parainfluenzae*
(iii) *H. parahaemolyticus*
(iv) *H. influenzae*
(v) *H. aegyptius*
(vi) *H. haemolyticus*

Serology

H. influenzae has six antigen types a–f, type b being the most common pathogen in children (i.e. under the age of 8). Serology does not apply to the differentiation of the other species.

Table III.6. Differentiation of haemophilus on X and V factor requirements.

	X factor only	V factor only	X and V factor
H. ducreyi	+	−	+
H. parainfluenzae	−	+	+
H. parahaemolyticus	−	+	+
H. influenzae	−	−	+
H. aegyptius	−	−	+
H. haemolyticus	−	−	+

Chapter 31
Bordetella

Bordetella belong to the family *Brucellaceae* and are the cause of whooping cough. Bordetella are non-motile Gram negative bacilli which grow anaerobically, are catalase variable, and oxidase positive. They do not grow on basal media, and are not biochemically active. They require neither X nor V factors for growth, but need special media for isolation. They are small Gram negative bacilli 1 μ in length. They are very definitely temperature dependent, i.e. any specimen should be received in the laboratory within 2 hours of collection, or else a Stuart or Amies Trans-Cul® swab should be used. See Chapter 4—the cough plate.

Cultural Characteristics

They grow on Bordet-Gengou's media for primary isolation and require 2–4 days at 37°C. Then the appear as small pearl-like colonies with a metallic sheen about 1 mm in diameter.

Diagnosis

Diagnosis is based on serology, and includes 3 species.

    (i) *B. pertussis* (continued viability at low temperature).

    (ii) *B. parapertussis*

    (iii) *B. bronchiseptica*

These can be determined biochemically as is shown in Table III.7.

Table III.7. Differentiation of Bordetella.

	Catalase	Urease	Aggln. with phase 1 sera
B. pertussis	−	−	+
B. parapertussis	+	+	−
B. bronchiseptica	+	+	+

Serology

Freshly isolated strains have 3 serotypes, 1, 2, 3, i.e. when using single factor absorbed sera.

Chapter 32
Brucella

Brucella is a Gram negative cocco-bacillus which is aerobic and non-motile; some species require 8–10 per cent CO_2 for growth. Catalase positive, urease positive, oxidase positive or negative, the species does not ferment sugars, and is non-capsulated and non-sporing. They grow better on enriched media, but only as small colonies 1 mm in diameter.

The three main species are classified according to the animal host, but man is also susceptible.

Classification

See Table III.8.

Table III.8. Differentiation of Brucella.

	B. abortus	B. suis	B. melitensis
Chief host	Cow	Pig	Goat, sheep
CO_2 requirement	+	−	−
Growth in serum thionin 1/30,000	−	+	+
Agar with basic fuchsin 1/25,000	+	−	+
Methyl violet 1/50,000	+	−	+
H_2S production	+ +	+ + +*	− (or slight)
Urease activity	120 min	15–30 min	Variable
Antigenically react as	B. abortus	B. abortus	B. melitensis

* Danish strains do not produce H_2S.

Diagnosis

Diagnosis is made from repeated blood culture from suspected patients, using Castaneda's blood culture medium with incubation under CO_2. The cultures should be kept for as long as 6 weeks before being discarded, but only about 30 per cent of cases produce positive blood cultures.

Serology

A more reliable indication of disease is by the use of agglutination tests, antibodies can be detected as soon as 7–10 days after the onset of infection. Prozone phenomena may be seen with high titres, and when this occurs, or when a negative result is obtained the test must be repeated using the modified Coombs technique. (Wilson & Merrifield,* 1951). Cross agglutination occurs within the species. False positive agglutination may occur in patients immunized against cholera, and those people who have antibodies to *Francisella tularensis*. All positive agglutinations should be checked by the 2 mercapto-ethanol method.

* Wilson, M. M. & Merrifield, E. V. O. (1951) The Anti-globulin (Coombs) Test in Brucellosis. *Lancet*, **ii**, 913.

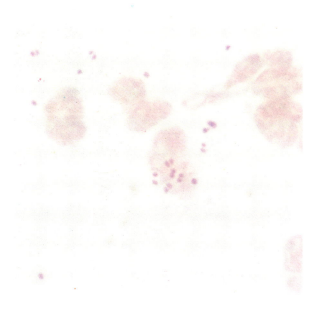

Fig. III.44. Neisseria gonorrhoeae on Gram stain. Gonococcal pus. Note that many of the *N. gonorrhoeae* are extracellular. × 3340.

Chapter 33
Neisseria

The *Neisseria* are Gram negative oval-shaped cocci usually occurring in pairs with their axis vertical (i.e. kidney-shaped). They are approximately 1 μ in diameter, non-motile, non-sporing and non-capsulated. They are both catalase and oxidase positive, and strictly aerobic (occasionally only with CO_2, e.g. the Gonococcus). If biochemically active, it is by oxidation. Pathogenic species require specially enriched media and under the microscope with Gram stain are found both as intracellular and extracellular organisms, more often the latter. Fig. III.44 shows a picture of gonococcal pus.

Cultural Characteristics

Pathogenic members of this genus, viz. *N. gonorrhoeae* and *N. meningitidis*, both show similar colonies on Thayer Martin (TM) medium with its added constituents. Chocolate agar (CA) is no longer used for diagnosis of *Neisseria* infections. Using 8–10 per cent CO_2 (Gas Pak® System) and incubation for 48 hours at 37°C similar translucent colonies are produced. They are 2–3 mm in size with a slightly roughened edge.

Diagnosis

Colonies of *N. gonorrhoeae* and *N. meningitidis* react strongly to the oxidase reagent whereas

Fig. III.45. Positive oxidase test on N. gonorrhoeae. A few drops of the oxidase reagent have been run over the surface of a Thayer Martin plate, and the gonococcus is oxidase positive, as shown by becoming purple after 10–30 seconds.

Fig. III.46. Biochemical reactions of N. gonorrhoeae. *N. gonorrhoeae* on glucose, maltose, and sucrose human serum sugars. After incubation the gonococcus has fermented the glucose on the left (as indicated by a change in colour of the indicator from pink to yellow), but neither the maltose nor sucrose.

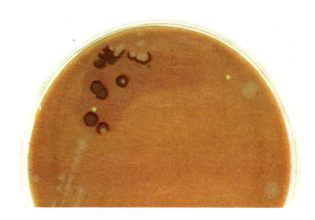

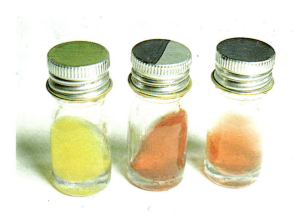

other non-pathogenic Neisseria become oxidase-positive quite slowly. This is well shown in Fig. III.45, and Fig. III.46 shows the classical sugar reactions of *N. gonorrhoeae*.

Further differentiation between the species can be made by the biochemical activity of organisms in glucose, maltose and sucrose, this may be a very important medico-legal point (see Table III.9).

Table III.9. Biochemical reactions of Neisseria

	Glucose	Maltose	Sucrose
N. catarrhalis	−	−	−
N. gonorrhoea	+(+acid)	−	−
N. meningitidis	+(+acid)	+(+acid)	−
N. pharyngis	+(+acid)	+(+acid)	+(+acid)

Serology

N. meningitidis may be serologically grouped into four main types (A–D). Group A is the most common cause of meningococcal meningitis, but more recently Groups B and C are being seen in some epidemics. *N. gonorrhoeae* is capable of being grouped into four biotypes (T1–T4) but in the main they are a heterogeneous group.

The Gonococcal Complement Fixation Test (GCFT) is used by some to prove the diagnosis of gonorrhoea. It is unreliable. It may be positive where the patient has not had gonorrhoea (past or present) but on the contrary may be negative in the case of a patient with either obvious acute or chronic gonorrhoea.

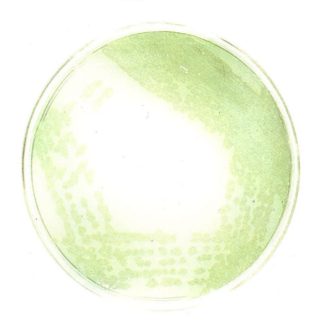

Fig. III.47. P. aeruginosa on nutrient agar. The characteristic green diffusible pigment and the metallic sheen can be seen.

Chapter 34
Pseudomonas, Leofflerella

Pseudomonas are Gram negative bacilli which are motile, catalase positive, oxidase positive, non-capsulated which grow aerobically. They are biochemically active by oxidation (glucose only), and do not produce gas. They grow on basal media, frequently producing a diffusible yellow or green pigment. There are more than 140 species in this genus, but the main one pathogenic to man is *Pseudomonas aeruginosa* (*P. pyocyanea*). They are ubiquitious in nature, and *P. aeruginosa* is often 'pathogenic'. It is an 'opportunist' in urinary tract infections, wound infections (particularly burns), respiratory tract infections, and also in patients on mechanical respirators and acute leukaemics, and other patients who are being given immunosuppressive drugs. *P.*

aeruginosa is also found in the intestinal tract of man and animals.

P. aeruginosa is the same size as the *Proteus spp.* but has fewer flagella, and these are polar in situation.

CULTURAL CHARACTERISTICS

On basal agar the organism appears as rough colonies, often with a metallic sheen, approximately 3 mm in diameter. The organism has a characteristic musty odour, and there is generally a diffusable pigment. On MacConkey agar it appears as a pale colony often with a green pigment. This is also well seen on NA (see Fig. III.47).

Diagnosis is made on the typical cultural characteristics, i.e. pigmentation and rapid oxidase test. (If necessary the oxidation-fermentation test using glucose can be performed.)

Serology has been found to have little application, although some 12 serological types have been distinguished.

Pyocine typing is used for epidemological pur-

poses, this is similar to colicine typing. At least 37 different types have been recognized.

Leofflerella

This genus includes the organism *P. pseudomallei*, because it gives a positive oxidase reaction and has polar flagella. This organism can present as indolent skin ulcers, or as a pyrexia of unknown origin (PUO), liver abscess or generally disseminated abscesses following septicaemia, and so is an important pathogen when it occurs, e.g. in S.E. Asia and Northern Australia.

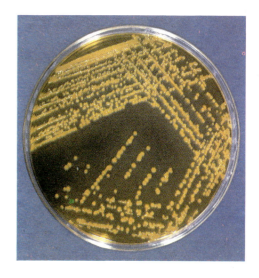

Fig. III.48. V. cholerae on TCBS agar. The organism has been plated out onto TCBS agar from an alkaline peptone water. *V. cholerae* grow as yellow colonies against the dark green background of the medium.

Table III.10. Differentiation between *V. cholerae* and *V. cholerae* biotype *El Tor*

Species	Cholera phage IV	Polymyxin B	Direct haemagglutination of chicken RBC
V. cholerae	Sensitive	Sensitive	Negative
V. cholerae biotype *El Tor*	Resistant	Resistant	Positive

Chapter 35
Vibrio and Spirillum

The vibrios are of the family *Spirillaceae*. They are Gram negative bacilli usually curved, motile, non-capsulated catalase positive, and oxidase positive. Aerobic or facultatively anaerobic, they are biochemically active by fermentation, but gas is not produced and arginine is not hydrolyzed. Some members are pathogenic, others mere commensals or saprophytic, particularly in water.

Vibrio cholerae and Vibrio cholerae Biotype El Tor

These are small Gram negative curved bacilli approximately 2 μ × 0.5 μ in size which have a single polar flagellum. They grow over a wide temperature range, and the optimum pH is 8.5–9.2. On MacConkey Agar the colonies appear small and colourless, but on selective media for the isolation of *V. cholerae* (TCBS) cholera medium (Thiosulphate Citrate Bile-salts Sucrose agar) they grow as bright yellow colonies 3 mm in diameter (see Fig. III.48).

DIAGNOSIS

After 4 hours incubation in alkaline peptone broth the organisms demonstrate extremely rapid motility which stops when specific antigen is added. This test together with the characteristic growth on TCBS cholera agar, helps to complete the diagnosis of *V. cholerae*, but other tests are necessary (see Table III.10).

V. cholerae and *V. cholerae El Tor* biotype can be serologically differentiated from other vibrios, on the basis of the somatic antigen group 1(01), all other vibrios are not agglutinated by this antigen and are often called non-agglutinating vibrios (NAG). The two pathogenic biotypes may be further divided into two serological subtypes 'Inaba' and 'Ogawa', again based on separate somatic antigens.

Paired sera taken 10 days apart should show a significant rise in titre to check the bacteriological diagnosis.

Spirillum

Spirillum minus is the causative organism of rat-bite fever. It is a short rigid spiral-shaped organism about $4 \mu \times 0.5 \mu$, with regular coils. It is Gram negative, non-capsulated and is actively motile due to terminal flagella. It is easily seen under the dark-ground microscope, and stains well with Leishman's stain.

Culture of the organism has yet to be achieved.

DIAGNOSIS

Diagnosis can be made by microscopic examination of stained films from the exudate, lymph glands and occasionally the blood. Alternatively, the exudate may be injected IP into a guinea pig, which dies from the infection, when the organism can again be demonstrated in the blood using dark-ground microscopy.

Chapter 36
Enterobacteriaceae

The *Enterobacteriaceae* are organisms which are interrelated, and are mainly indistinguishable by Gram stain. Usually 3.5 $\mu \times 0.5$ μ in size, they are Gram negative, straight rods with rounded ends. Some genera are motile, and some possess capsules. All members of the family are biochemically active for glucose by fermentation, some with the production of gas. They also grow well on basal medium.

Some are normal inhabitants of the human intestinal tract, but both these and others may be pathogenic for man. Many of these organisms can also be isolated from wounds, sputum, CSF and blood.

Fig. III.49. Gram stain of E. coli.
The *E. coli* appear as Gram negative
bacilli. × 4342.

**Fig. III.50. E. coli on MacConkey
agar.** The *E. coli* after incubation appear
as large pink lactose fermenting colonies.
Small pale colonies can also be seen, these
are non-lactose fermenting organisms.

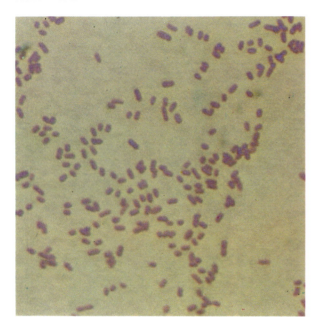

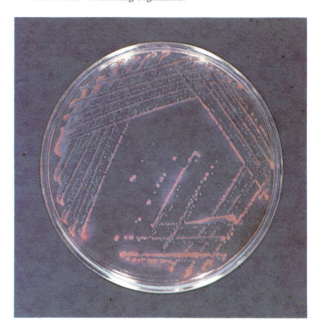

Escherichia coli

E. coli are Gram negative bacilli, which are
motile, catalase positive, oxidase negative, and
facultatively anaerobic; they are biochemically
active by fermentation, usually with the production of gas. They are unable to utilize citrate as
the carbon source, and are also KCN negative.
They are ubiquitous in nature and are commonly
found in the intestine of both man and animals.
They are motile, with peritrichous flagella.

Under the microscope the rods are 3 μ × 0.5 μ
in size and Gram negative (see Fig. III.49 which
shows the typical microscopical appearance of *E.
coli*).

CULTURAL CHARACTERISTICS

E. coli grows rapidly at 37°C on basal agar. After
18–24 hours the colonies appear approximately
3 mm in diameter, and are opaque, convex and
possess an entire edge. On MacConkey's agar
they appear as red colonies 2–3 mm in diameter
(see Fig. III.50). In this picture *E. coli* appear
as red, large colonies, but there is a mixture with
non-lactose fermenting organisms.

On blood agar they may produce some haemolysis around the colony.

DIAGNOSIS

Diagnosis is based on the different biochemical
activities of the organism to a wide range of

Table III.11. The IMVEC test

Genus	Motility	Indole	Methyl-red (MR)	Voges-Proskauer (VP)	Eijkman	Citrate
		I	M	V	E	C
Escherichia	+	+	+	−	+	−
Citrobacter	+	−	+	−	+	+
Klebsiella	−	−	−	+	−	+

tests. More than 95 per cent ferment lactose, and are usually characterized by the IMVEC test initially (see Table III.11).

Some strains however, may be atypical and do not fall into any specific group.

SEROLOGY

The antigenicity of the genus is based on the presence of various O, H and K antigens. The most interesting of these is the K type of antigen—a group of antigens designated L, A or B on the basis of their differing physical characteristics. These K antigens occur as capsules or envelopes and like other surface antigens may prevent agglutination with the homologous somatic antisera. Virulence appears to be associated with the K antigen, impeding phagocytosis. Its role may be similar to that of the Vi antigen in *S. typhi*. Most of the virulent strains appear to be associated with the B type antigen. About 16 different O-serotypes have been associated with gastroenteritis.

Citrobacter freundii

C. freundii are motile, catalase positive, oxidase negative Gram negative bacilli which are facultatively anaerobic. They are biochemically active by fermentation (usually with gas production). *C. freundii* is able to utilize citrate as the carbon source; it is KCN positive.

Some of these Gram negative rods are larger than usual, being 3–4 μ × 1–0.5 μ in size.

CULTURAL CHARACTERISTICS

C. freundii grows rapidly at 37°C on basal agar. After 18–24 hours the colonies appear approximately 4 mm in diameter, and are glistening and mucoid with an entire edge. On MacConkey's agar they appear as mucoid red colonies 3 mm in diameter.

DIAGNOSIS

Diagnosis is based on the different biochemical activities of the organism over a wide range of tests, and are usually characterized by the IMVEC test (see Table III.11).

SEROLOGY

Little is known of the serology of this group of organisms, but there appear to be two distinct types.

Klebsiella

Klebsiella are non-motile, catalase positive, oxidase negative Gram negative bacilli which are facultatively anaerobic. They are biochemically active by fermentation (usually with the production of gas) and further are capable of utilization

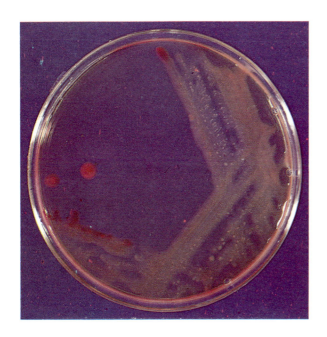

Fig. III.51. K. pneumoniae on Mac-Conkey agar. These organisms after incubation appear as large pink, glistening mucoid colonies.

of citrate, and are KCN positive, and may hydrolyze urea. Many strains are ubiquitous, and they are often encapsulated.

Under the microscope they are similar to the other members of the *Enterobacteriaceae* family, but a capsule may be seen.

CULTURAL CHARACTERISTICS

Colonies on basal agar are usually 4 mm in diameter, and are mucoid (due to extracellular slime). The colonies tend to coalesce. On MacConkey's agar the colonies are pink, mucoid and glistening (see Fig. III.51).

SPECIES

Six species exist and are distinguished by their biochemical reactions, but many authors refer only to three species, viz. the first three below:

1 *K. aerogenes*
2 *K. pneumoniae*
3 *K. edwardsii*
4 *K. atlantae*
5 *K. ozaenae*
6 *K. rhinoscleromatis*

Diagnosis is based on the biochemical tests, usually the IMVEC test (see Table III.11).

SEROLOGY

In addition to somatic antigens, most strains possess K (capsular), and M (mucoid) antigens, in each species both are identical. These antigens are used in typing as they mask the O antigen—the 'capsular swelling' reaction reveals more than 72 serotypes (similar to that of the Pneumococcus).

Shigella

These Gram negative rods are non-motile, non-capsulated, catalase positive and oxidase negative, they are also facultatively anaerobic and biochemically active by fermentation, but usually without gas production. They do not utilize citrate, are KCN negative, and H_2S is not produced. They grow on basal agar.

CULTURAL CHARACTERISTICS

Growth is similar to that of other members of the family on basal agar, but on MacConkey's agar, desoxycholate agar or Salmonella-Shigella agar, they appear as pale colonies (i.e. non-

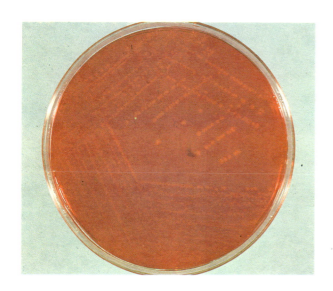

Fig. III.52. Shigella on XLD media.
The organisms appear as red colonies.

lactose fermenting) after incubation at 37°C for 18 hours. On XLD media (xylose, lysine, desoxycholate agar) they appear as red colonies. This latter medium is an ideal one for Shigella (see Fig. III.52).

DIAGNOSIS

Diagnosis is based on biochemical activity. Four species are concerned in this genus:

viz.   *S. dysenteriae*   (Group A)
       S. flexneri   (Group B)
       S. boydii   (Group C)
       S. sonnei   (Group D)

The biochemical distinction between Groups ABC and D is that the latter is both ONPG* and mannitol positive, whereas Groups AB and C are all ONPG negative.

SEROLOGY

However, each species has a number of serotypes, based on their somatic antigens, and the species can be determined by group specific agglutination, as can individual serotypes.

There are 10 specific types in Group A, 6 serotypes in Group B, 15 serotypes in Goup C, and 1 serotype in Group D. (Group D can be further subdivided by colicine typing into 17 types.)

* ONPG is orthonitrophenyl-β-D galacto-pyranoside which turns bright yellow by the production of -o-nitro-phenol when the test is positive.

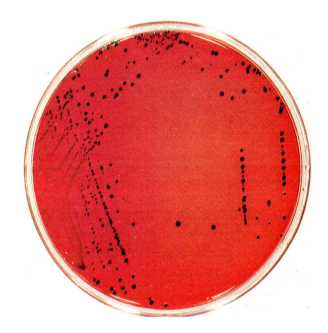

Fig. III.53. S. typhimurium on XLD media. The organisms appear as large red colonies with a black centre which tends to make the whole colony appear black.

Salmonella

These Gram negative bacilli are usually motile and catalase positive, but oxidase negative, also they are facultatively anaerobic. They are biochemically active by fermentation usually producing gas. Growth occurs on basal media and they utilize citrate as a carbon source, are KCN negative and usually produce H_2S. They are ubiquitous in nature and there are more than 1000 serotypes within the genus.

CULTURAL CHARACTERISTICS

Growth similar to other members of the family occurs on basal agar, but on MacConkey's agar, desoxycholate agar and Salmonella-Shigella agar, *Salmonella* appear as pale colonies with an entire edge. On XLD media they appear as red colonies with a black centre (see Fig. III.53).

DIAGNOSIS

Diagnosis is based on biochemical activity, fermentation of mannitol and glucose with the production of gas, and the production of H_2S. Also the demonstration of motility is an important character dependent on the flagella present on organisms of this group.

Table III.12. Serology of the common Salmonellae.

Group	Example of serotype	Somatic antigens	Specific antigen	Flagella antigens Phase I	Flagella antigens Phase II
A	*S. paratyphi* A	1, 2, 12	2	a	—
B	*S. paratyphi* B	4, 5, 12	4	b	1, 2
	S. typhimurium	1, 4, 5, 12	4	i	1, 2
C$_1$	*S. choleraesuis*	6, 7	7	c	1, 5
	S. thompson	6, 7	7	k	1, 5
C$_2$	*S. bovis-morbificans*	6, 8	8	r	1, 5
	S. newport	6, 8	8	e h	1, 2
D	*S. typhi*	9, 12 Vi	9	d	—
	S. enteriditis	1, 9, 12	9	gm	—
E$_4$	*S. senftenberg*	1, 3, 1, 9	19	g s t	—

Other additional groups also exist.

SEROLOGY

Further identification is made on the basis of specific somatic and flagella antigens⋆ (see Table III.12).

Bacteriophage may be used on the serotypes isolated from an outbreak of food poisoning, e.g. *S. typhimurium*, so that the phage type of the isolates from the patients may be matched from the infected food or from a suspected animal source, therefore this is an important epidemiological tool.

⋆ A few salmonella possess a third antigen occurring on the surface and designated the Vi antigen; when present it masks agglutination with 0 antisera, but in the case of *S. typhi* the specific Vi antigen is diagnostic.

Proteus

The members of this genus are motile, non-capsulated, catalase positive, oxidase negative, facultatively anaerobic and biochemically active by fermentation, usually with the production of gas. They hydrolyse urea rapidly, and are phenylalanine and KCN positive. They are ubiquitous in nature and may occur as pathogens in wounds, respiratory or urinary tract infections and in other sites. Infection may be exogenous or endogenous in origin.

The organisms are similar to other Enterobacteriaceae, but tend to pleomorphism under the microscope.

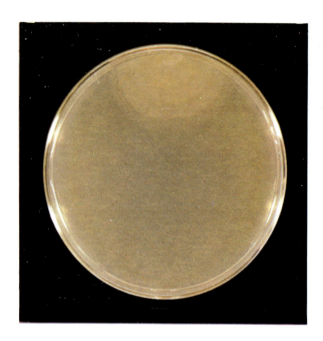

Fig. III.54. Swarming of Proteus on basal agar. Proteus has been inoculated by a straight wire on the top of the plate. Proteus can be seen as swarming over the plate in a wave-like motion.

CULTURAL CHARACTERISTICS

These are similar to other members of the family with the exception that some species swarm on basal agar (see Fig. III.54). Swarming is due to vigorous motility, and may be inhibited by various means such as bile salts, etc. On MacConkey's agar or desoxycholate agar they appear as pale yellow colonies, on XLD agar they appear as yellow colonies.

DIAGNOSIS

Four species or biotypes exist within this genus, and can be differentiated biochemically, viz.

Proteus vulgaris
Proteus mirabilis
Proteus morganii
Proteus rettgeri

Most clinical isolates are *P. mirabilis*, other species are generally highly antibiotic resistant (Table III.13).

SEROLOGY

P. vulgaris and *P. mirabilis* between them have been found to have 119 serotypes which can be recognized on the basis of H and O antigens.

Certain strains of proteus have antigens in common with the rickettsiae; X19 and XK, O antigens have been used in the Weil-Felix test

Table III.13. Biochemical differentiation of Proteus spp.

	Gelatin liquefaction	Maltose	Mannitol	H_2S production	Indole production	Swarming at 37°C on NA
P. vulgaris	+	AG	−	+	+	+
P. mirabilis	+	−	−	+	−	+
P. morganii	−	−	−	−	+	−
P. rettgeri	−	−	AG	−	+	−

for the diagnosis of typhus fevers. OX19 is positive in European typhus (*R. prowazeki*), OXK is positive in scrub typhus (*R. tsutsugamushi*).

Chapter 37
Pasteurella, Yersinia and Francisella

Pasteurella falls into the group *Yersinia*; they are small Gram negative bacilli which may be either motile or non-motile, are catalase positive, oxidase negative, and facultatively anaerobic. They are biochemically active by fermentation with gas production, and they ferment sucrose but do not grow on MacConkey's agar, e.g. *Pasteurella pestis* (*Y. pestis*).

The main pathogen in this group is *P. pestis* or more correctly *Y. pestis* which is a small cocco-bacillus, showing bipolar staining and pleomorphism. It is capsulated in fresh specimens from patients.

CULTURAL CHARACTERISTICS

Y. pestis grows best anaerobically at 27°C. It grows on basal agar, but large colonies are seen when blood or serum is added to the media. The colonies appear greyish, and are somewhat irregular in shape. *Y. pestis* is non-motile, and indole negative.

DIAGNOSIS

Diagnosis is made by staining the exudate from a bubo, or from sputum in pneumonic plague. The specimen is then stained with methylene blue, showing the characteristic small cocco-bacilli with bipolar staining—this is confirmed by culture onto BA, and by animal inoculation.

Both somatic and capsular antigens are serologically homogeneous in all strains.

The material is inoculated onto the nasal mucosa of guinea pigs or rats. In septicaemic plague the organisms may be found in blood culture or seen in smears from the spleen at post-mortem.

Francisella tularensis (Pasteurella tularensis)

The organism formerly known as *Pasteurella tularensis* is now classed in a separate genus, *Francisella*, and is the cause of tularaemia in man; it is similar to *Y. pestis* in size, and is also encapsulated, with a tendency to pleomorphism. It cannot be cultured on ordinary media, but requires a complex media containing egg yolk or pieces of sterile rabbit spleen, or alternatively the addition of blood, glucose and cystine.

Diagnosis is usually performed by inoculation of the exudate into guinea pigs or mice.

The patient's serum can be tested for agglutinating antibodies. There may however be a cross reaction with persons infected with *Brucella*.

Chapter 38
Bacteroides

The *Bacteroides* are Gram negative pleomorphic bacilli 2–3 μ long, non-sporing, which may be motile and are strict anaerobes. They are common inhabitants of the respiratory, intestinal and also the genital tract. They are biochemically active by fermentation.

The group can be subclassified according to biochemical activity, cultural characteristics and on specific morphology.

(i) *Bacteroides fragilis* is a small rod 2 μ × 0.5 μ often staining irregularly and frequently pleomorphic. It is a normal commensal in the intestine, and is the most common Gram negative anaerobic organism isolated from clinical material when strictly anaerobic conditions are applied in the laboratory.

(ii) *Bacteroides necrophorus* is a larger, pleomorphic filamentous organism. It has a central band which tends to stain less intensely than the rest of the rod.

(iii) Third, is a miscellaneous group including the following important species amongst many others:

(a) *B. melaninogenicus* which produces a black pigment on blood agar.

(b) *B. corrodens* whose colonies tend to dig into the agar.

DIAGNOSIS

The use of a selective media such as Willis and Hobbs agar for isolation is mandatory. Strictly anaerobic conditions must be maintained.

Fusobacterium fusiformis

This organism does not fit completely into the above classification. It stains poorly by Gram's method and is best stained by dilute carbol fuchsin for 10–15 minutes. In conjunction with *Borrelia vincentii* it is the causative agent of Vincent's angina. It is a strict anaerobe, but is easily seen under phase microscopy.

Chapter 39
Treponema and Borrelia

The genus Treponema consists of a large number of organisms but the only ones which are of medical importance are *Treponema pallidum* which causes syphilis, *T. pertenue* responsible for yaws and *T. carateum* which causes pinta.

Treponema pallidum is a tightly coiled helix 6–14 μ long by 0.1 μ wide, both ends are tapered and the organisms have 6–12 coils which are evenly distributed at 1 μ intervals. They are very motile, due to flexion and rotation of the whole cell from superficial fibrils. They do not stain with aniline dyes, and are best observed by dark-ground illumination microscopy, or they can be stained by Giemsa (24 hr method), or by silver impregnation. They are highly susceptible

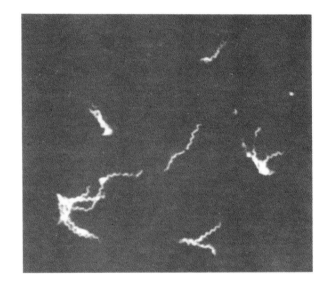

Fig. III.55. T. pallidum. Extracted from rabbit testes. The original photograph was of treponemes fluorescing in the FTA-ABS test × 4342.

to drying and mild heat (42°C), also they are cold sensitive and do not survive at 4°C for more than a few days, thus any specimen requires immediate investigation in the laboratory as no method is known for culture, but the organism is reproduced in the rabbit testis, scrotum or eye.

DIAGNOSIS

In primary and secondary lesions it is possible to obtain the spirochaetes directly by scraping the chancre or after aspirating fluid from a lesion in the secondary stage rash, and immediately searching for the organism under dark-ground illumination. The fluorescent antibody test is better in more experienced hands (Fig. III.55).

SEROLOGY

Various tests and their optimum times of performance are shown in Table III.14. A screening test, the RPR®★ (Rapid Plasma Reagin) test is available for serum and is very accurate.

Treponema pertenue

This species is indistinguishable from *T. pallidum* therefore the diagnostic procedures are the same, with cross-immunity between yaws (which it causes) and syphilis.

Treponema carateum

Also indistinguishable from *T. pallidum*; immunologically some difference exists because

★ Hynson, Westcott & Dunning, Inc., Baltimore, Maryland. 21201. U.S.A.

Table III.14. The serology of syphilis

Clinical stage Exposure and infection		Test(s)
10–90 days		
	3–4 weeks	
av. 21 days		
Primary chancre		FTA ABS
	1–2 weeks	Reagin tests, e.g.: VDRL, WR or Kahn test
	6–12 weeks	In varying order, but all positive by secondary stage
Secondary syphilis	{	RPCFT TPI TPHA
Latent syphilis	5–15 years	
Tertiary syphilis	{	FTA ABS } usually reactive TPI and TPHA} for life Reagin tests may become non-reactive

Key: FTA ABS   Absorbed Fluorescent Treponemal Antibody Test
     VDRL   Venereal Disease Research Laboratory Test
     WR   Wasserman Test
     RPCFT   Reiter Protein Complement Fixation Test
     TPI   *Treponema pallidum* Haemagglutination Test
     TPHA   *Treponema pallidum* Haemagglutination Test

patients with pinta may contract syphilis. Laboratory diagnosis is similar to that of syphilis.

Borrelia

Borrelia are long 20 μ × 0.3 μ motile, spirochaetes, with three to eight irregular spirals. They are Gram negative and non-sporing.

Two member species in this genus are human pathogens, one causing relapsing fever, *Borrelia recurrentis* (louse-borne relapsing fever), and the other *Borrelia duttoni* (tick-borne relapsing fever). Both are morphologically similar, but differ serologically. They are difficult to culture on artificial media, but animal inoculation in mice is useful for primary isolation. Blood films can be examined after staining with Leishman's stain or with dilute carbol fuchsin for 10–15 minutes. Dark-ground illumination may also be used. If the organism is not demonstrated by the above techniques, mice can be injected IP with the patient's blood. After 48 hours the organisms will be detectable in the animal's blood using the microscopic techniques described above.

BORRELIA VINCENTII

This organism in conjunction with *Fusobacterium fusiformis* (see Chapter 38) is the cause of Vincent's angina in humans.

The clinical diagnosis is made by taking scrap-

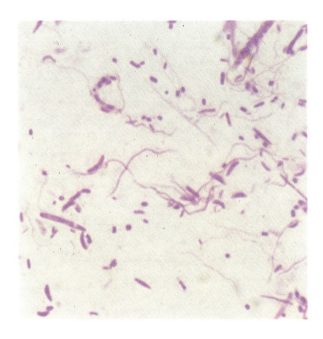

ings of the lesions and staining the smears with dilute carbol fuchsin where the typical picture of the two organisms can be seen. See Fig. III.56. But the diagnosis can also be surmised after examination under phase microscopy of scrapings from suspicious ulcers in the mouth of a patient.

Chapter 40
Leptospira

Leptospires are spiral organisms 6–20 μ long and 0.1 μ wide, the ends are usually hooked, and the coils are numerous and tightly packed together. They are motile by reversible spinning. They stain poorly with aniline dyes, but can be readily detected by dark-ground illumination and by silver impregnation stain, see Figs. III.57 and 58. They grow only on semi-solid agar containing rabbit serum, and the optimum temperature is 28°C–32°C, but growth is slow, particularly if primary isolation is attempted at 37°C, and 2–3 weeks may elapse before growth is obvious.

Diagnosis

Diagnosis can be confirmed if the leptospires

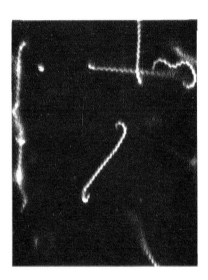

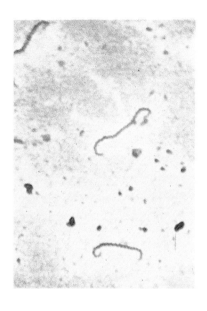

Fig. III.57 (left). Leptospires under dark-ground illumination. × 4342.

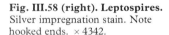

Fig. III.58 (right). Leptospires. Silver impregnation stain. Note hooked ends. × 4342.

are isolated from the blood, but they only appear in the peripheral blood during the first week of the disease. If the blood is collected during the first few days of illness and injected IP into a young guinea pig, blood is then collected by cardiac puncture and cultured.

The organisms may be present in the urine during the second week of illness and may continue to be excreted intermittently for 4–6 weeks and can be seen in the centrifuged deposit using dark-ground illumination, however the pH of the urine needs to be as nearly neutral as possible (pH 7) as the leptospires are very sensitive to acidic conditions, therefore the urine should be inspected immediately after voiding.

Antibodies appear after the first week, but tend to decline during the second to the fourth week. Since resident agglutinating antibodies may remain for many years, a rise in antibody titre of paired sera is required. This can be done using a rapid macroscopic slide agglutination test.

Many species of leptospira exist, but the pathogenic species has been named *Leptospira interrogans*. Weil's Disease is usually due to the serotype *icterohaemorrhagiae* and the course may vary from mild to fatal. Other serotypes may also cause spirochaetal jaundice in other parts of the world, e.g. *australis* and *bataviae*.

SECTION IV
MYCOLOGY

Introduction

Until recently fungal diseases were thought to be largely seen in superficial infections and their diagnosis was generally considered confined to dermatologists. Current experience shows that active systemic mycoses, or evidence of such previous disease in healthy individuals, is not uncommon. The survival of patients treated with immunosuppresive drugs has also contributed to the number of active fungal diseases.

This section deals with fungal diseases that are commonly seen in man. To compare their incidence with bacterial disease would be unreal, but it is important to realize they may be a possible causative factor in disease and thus be able to recognize them in the laboratory.

Also, the headings in parts of this section relate

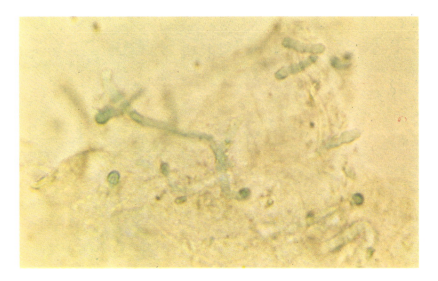

Fig. IV.1. Malassezia furfur. A 10 per cent KOH preparation of skin scales showing clusters of round thick-walled budding cells (3–8 μ) in diameter, together with thick short mycelial elements. × 1280.

Chapter 41
Tinea Versicolor (Malassezia furfur)

to the diseases caused by the particular fungi or species of fungi. This has been done deliberately because most people know fungi by the name of the disease they cause rather than the name of the fungus itself.

The instruments required for obtaining specimens for fungal culture are shown in Fig. II.25. The stain normally used for microscopy in mycology is lactophenal blue.

Tinea versicolor is a superficial fungal infection of the skin seen in all parts of the world. It is caused by *M. furfur*. The fungus fluoresces yellow under Wood's light. It is seen in the horny layers of the skin, from which it can be obtained by skin scrapings. In the scrapings or scales it appears as round budding cells with mycelial elements. Fig. IV.1.

Culture of scales on special media has resulted in a growth of *Pityrosporum orbiculare* which some consider identical to *M. furfur*. In most people's hands, however, culture is usually unsuccessful. Direct staining techniques are reliable whether Gram, periodic-acid Schiff or Giemsa are used. In KOH specimens the typical organisms are short, thickish hyphal elements of

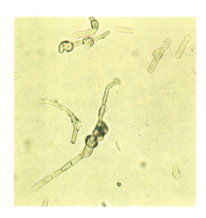

Fig. IV.2. Cladosporium werneckii.
A lactophenol blue preparation from a Sabouraud culture of epidermal scrapings from a patient with tinea nigra palmaris. Note the branched, septate hyphae and some also showing arthrospore-like structures as well. The hyphae are usually 1.5–3 μ in diameter. × 1336.

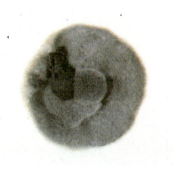

Fig. IV.3. Growth of Cladosporium werneckii. The surface shows a slow growing glabrous colony at 14 days at 30°C, Sabouraud's agar. The olive green colony shows a heaped-up central growth and a degree of surface folding with an entire greyish-black edge. Note the relative absence of aerial mycelial growth at this temperature.

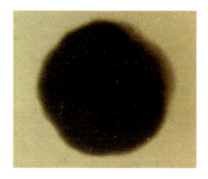

Fig. IV.4. Cladosporium werneckii (Underside). The underside is smooth and greyish-black in colour.

Chapter 42
Tinea Nigra (Cladosporium werneckii and C. mansonii)

various shapes and sizes. Sometimes these are straight but more often are contoured and irregular, occasionally being S- or V-shaped. Round spores, often in grapelike clusters are generally the rule—their diameter varies and on occasion there are budding extrusions.

This is another superficial mycosis seen in tropical and subtropical regions. The genus *Cladosporium* is said to be synonymous with *Hormodendron*. The palms are most frequently involved, but the disease may also affect the thorax, neck and soles.

After treatment of the specimen with KOH the fungus appears as pigmented, light brown to dark green, branching septate hyphae 1.5–3 μ in diameter (see Fig. IV.2). Long flexed hyphae and swollen closely septate fragments appear as chlamydospores.

The fungus grows slowly on Sabouraud's agar as a black, shiny yeast-like colony up to 15 days when the colour changes to dark green and aerial mycelia develop (Fig. IV.3, and IV.4).

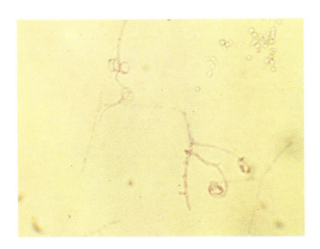

Fig. IV.5. Trichophyton mentagrophytes. Characteristic preparation showing coiled, spiral, serpentine hyphae and clusters of clavate microconidia, some borne laterally on the hyphae. × 334.

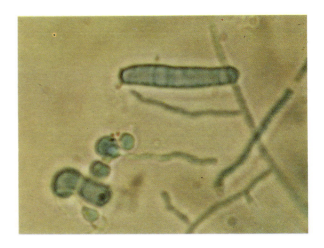

Fig. IV.6. Trichophyton rubrum. This preparation shows the characteristic long and slender hyphae of *T. rubrum*. Note the tear-shaped microconidia and thin-walled slender, cigar-shaped macroconidia. × 668.

Chapter 43
Dermatophytoses

Members of *Trichophyton*, *Microsporum* and *Epidermophyton spp*. make up the dermatophytes. Microscopically the common finding in these species is abundant microconidia. The appearance of the longish hyphae varies from serpentine in *T. mentagrophytes* to long and slender in *T. rubrum* (Figs. IV.5 and IV.6).

Trichophyton Species

The different cultural characteristics are well seen on Sabouraud's or mycobiotic media and are shown in the following figures:

Fig. IV.7. *T. mentagrophytes* (Surface)
  IV.8. *T. mentagrophytes* (Underside)
  IV.9. *T. rubrum* (Surface)
  IV.10. *T. rubrum* (Underside)
  IV.11. *T. violaceum* (Surface)
  IV.12. *T. violaceum* (Underside)
  IV.13. *T. schoenleinii* (Surface)
  IV.14. *T. schoenleinii* (Underside)
  IV.15. *T. tonsurans* (Surface)
  IV.16. *T. tonsurans* (Underside)
  IV.17. *T. verrucosum* (Surface)
  IV.18. *T. verrucosum* (Underside)

Tinea capitis is caused by *T. mentagrophytes*, *T. violaceum*, *T. schoenleinii*, and *T. tonsurans*, in fact by any of the dermatophytes except *T. concentricum*. Tinea barbae is caused mainly by *T. mentagrophytes* or *T. verrucosum* and only occasionally by *T. rubrum*, *T. violaceum* and

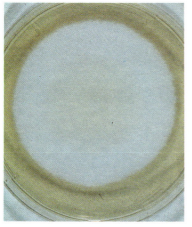

IV.7

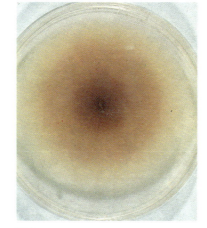

IV.8

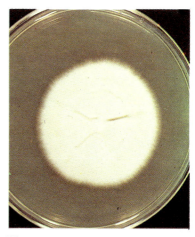

IV.9

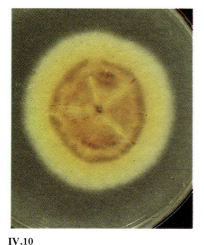

IV.10

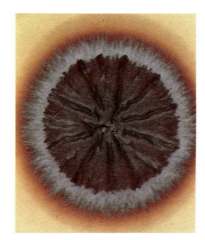

IV.11

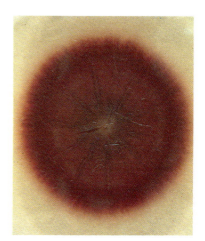

IV.12

Fig. IV.7. T. mentagrophytes
(Surface). Fast-growing colony on
the surface of Sabouraud's agar showing
a white central papilla with a ring of
creamy, buff, downy surface growth with
a white fluffy fringed periphery.

Fig. IV.8. T. mentagrophytes
(Underside). The underside is notable
for a dark brown centre which diminishes
in colour almost to cream as the
periphery is reached.

Fig. IV.9. T. rubrum (Surface). The
surface thallus may be either fluffy or
granular—two distinct types. The
colour ranges from white to pinkish red
and the colony develops a floccose or
cottony to powdery appearance. In this

instance, the downy colony shows a
raised central white tuft with radiating
cream to lime green undulated broad
folds advancing towards a white fringed
edge.

Fig. IV.10. T. rubrum (Underside).
The radiating ridges cutting across the
colony can be seen clearly. The centre of
the thallus is a light reddish brown and
colour deepens to a dotted brown ring
which is encircled by another outer dark
brown ring. Colour remains a light
brownish yellow for the rest of the
colony.

Fig. IV.11. T. violaceum (Surface).
The photo shows a slow-growing wax-
like thallus. The colonial surface has rows

of deep radially arranged folds and
ridges. The colour begins as deep violet
ranging through to a lilac fringed
periphery with submerged growth.

Fig. IV.12. T. violaceum (Underside).
The underside shows deep ridges
radiating from the centre. The colour
is dark red to purplish brown and
accentuates the fringed periphery.

Dermatophytoses 121

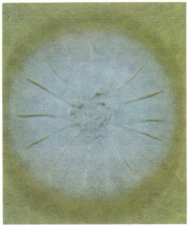

IV.13

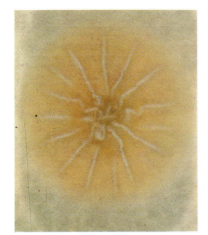

IV.14

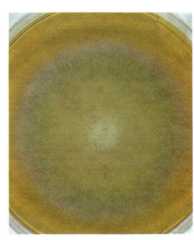

IV.15

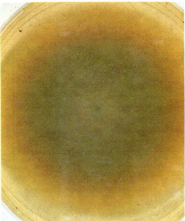
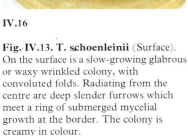

IV.16

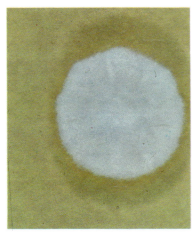

IV.17

IV.18

Fig. IV.13. T. schoenleinii (Surface). On the surface is a slow-growing glabrous or waxy wrinkled colony, with convoluted folds. Radiating from the centre are deep slender furrows which meet a ring of submerged mycelial growth at the border. The colony is creamy in colour.

Fig. IV.14. T. schoenleinii (Underside). The underside shows radiating and slightly twisted ridges. These are characteristic and well shown. The colour is pale buff.

Fig. IV.15. T. tonsurans (Surface). The colonial surface is variable showing colours from white, yellow, buff, brown to red. The texture varies from velvety to powdery and the surface pattern may be flat or show different degrees of radial folds. In the picture shown the flat powdery thallus is buff in colour with a central papilla and a pinkish brown periphery.

Fig. IV.16. T. tonsurans (Underside). The underside shows a small dark brown centre surrounded by a small pale orange ring of growth. The colour of the colony deepens to brownish-red towards the advancing edge.

Fig. IV.17. T. verrucosum (Surface). The surface slow-growing thallus is small, white and downy—it is moderately folded with narrow radiating depressions. The colony has a central tuft which is raised, but the periphery is flat.

Fig. IV.18. T. verrucosum (Underside). The underside of the colony is light buff in colour with the impression of radiating furrows visible.

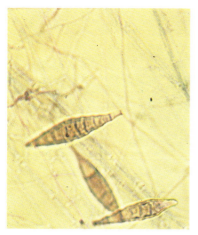

IV.19

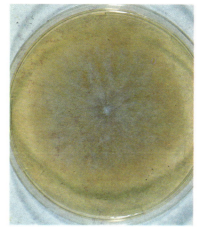

IV.20

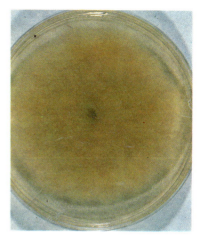

IV.21

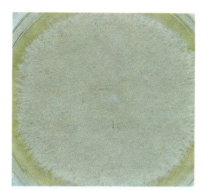

IV.22

Fig. IV.19. Microsporum canis. This preparation shows the typical thick-walled multiseptate spindle-shaped macroconidia of *M. canis* under the microscope; typical long and short hyphae are also visible. × 668.

Fig. IV.20. M. canis (Surface). The cottony spreading aerial mycelial surface growth is easily recognizable after 7 days incubation. The colour of the colony varies from white, light buff to golden yellow. The thallus has a small central papilla.

Fig. IV.21. M. canis (Underside). There is a small brownish centre with light brown colour diffusing through the downy colour.

Fig. IV.22. M. gypseum (Surface). On the surface can be seen a rapidly growing powdery colony. Its colour varies from white to fawn brown. The surface is floccose with an irregularly fringed edge.

Microsporum canis. The common causative agents of tinea corporis or circinata in ring-worm of the non-hairy skin are *T. mentagrophytes*, *T. rubrum*, *M. canis* and *M. audouinii*.

Tinea cruris in its various types is due to *T. mentagrophytes*, *Epidermophyton floccosum* or *T. rubrum*. The same fungi are the common causes of tinea of the feet and hands. Hairs infected by *T. schoenleinii* fluoresce under Wood's light.

Microsporum Species

These have characteristic multiseptate macroconidia microscopically. *M. canis* typically is spindle shaped. Hyphae are always slender and straight, Fig. IV.19. Growth is either on Sabouraud's or mycobiotic media. Typical colonies are shown in the following figures.

Fig. IV.20.　*Microsporum canis* (Surface)
　　IV.21.　*Microsporum canis* (Underside)
　　IV.22.　*Microsporum gypseum* (Surface)
　　IV.23.　*Microsporum gypseum* (Underside)

In addition to the diseases mentioned earlier caused by this group of fungi, *M. gypseum* is responsible for onychomycosis. *M. audouinii* is another less common member of this species. *M. gypseum* is also the only one of this three not to fluoresce under Wood's light.

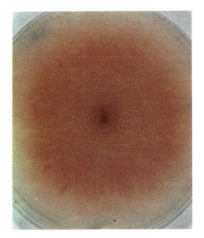

IV.23

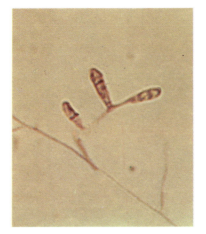

IV.24

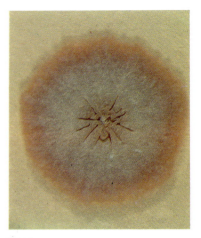

IV.25

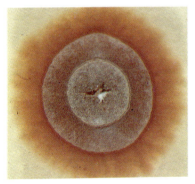

IV.26

Fig. IV.23. M. gypseum (Underside). The underside shows a yellow-brown colony surrounding a small buff central area. The periphery is irregular.

Fig. IV.24. Epidermophyton floccosum. Needle mount preparation showing characteristic smooth, thin-walled clavate macroconidia with long slender hyphae. × 668.

Fig. IV.25. E. floccosum (Surface). The surface is very characteristic. *E. floccosum* is slow-growing and gives an olive green colony, slightly powdery in texture with a suede-like appearance. The colony is centrally folded with small but sharp radiating grooves reaching out towards a fringed periphery.

Fig. IV.26. E. floccosum (Underside). The cinnamon-brown colony gives a hard, dry crusty appearance. The central papilla and its surrounding area are conspicuously demarcated by two rings of deep cuts.

Epidermophyton Species

Epidermophyton floccosum is the only common member of the species which is encountered clinically. Microscopically these are character-istically smooth, thin-walled, club-shaped mac-roconidia, with straight slender hyphae (Fig. IV.24).

Culture on Sabouraud's medium shows the fungus to be slow growing (15 days), olive green in colour and powdery; older cultures become enfolded and suede-like.

Fig. IV.25. *Epidermophyton floccosum*
    (Surface)
 IV.26. *Epidermophyton floccosum*
    (Underside)

This fungus causes tinea cruris or pedis and is also a cause of onychomycosis.

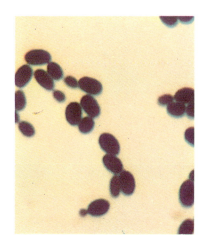

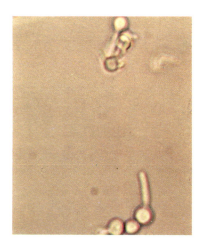

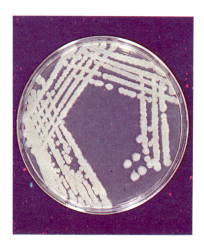

Fig. IV.27. Candida albicans. A Gram stained preparation shows the typical oval Gram positive organisms, some of which have budding forms arising from the parent cell. × 4342.

Fig. IV.28. Candida albicans. The characteristic germ tube formation can be seen as long slender elongated protoplasmic protrusions. × 1336.

Fig. IV.29. Candida albicans. Growth at 37°C for 48 hours on Sabouraud's agar shows smooth creamy-white raised colonies with an entire edge. The colonies are approximately 2 mm in diameter.

Chapter 44
Candidiasis

There are at least 68 members of the *Candida* spp. The common human pathogen is *Candida albicans*. Unfortunately it is a commensal in the mouth, vagina and gut, and is often found harmlessly on the skin. This makes the differentiation of disease from the commensal state difficult and thus diagnosis remains essentially a quantitative matter.

Occasionally the fungus may cause disease of the skin (particularly fingernails), mouth, vagina, bowel, or rarely it may present as septicaemia, endocarditis, meningitis, lung abscess or other forms of metastatic disease.

The fungus appears on Gram stain as a small oval 3–9 μ × 3.5–12 μ thin-walled yeast, sometimes budding. Mycelial elements occur and budding cells may be attached to the hyphae at the points of constriction (Fig. IV.27).

Proof of *C. albicans* infection is by the production of germ tubes when the isolate is incubated at 37°C in 10 per cent human serum for two hours (Fig. IV.28).

Culture is best performed on MA (plus gentamicin) although other workers use Sabouraud's agar. Growth occurs in 24–48 hours at 37°C and is characterized by a very marked smell of brewer's yeast. The colonies grow almost as well on basal as enriched media but not on selective media (Fig. IV.29). They appear as creamy, medium-sized moist to dull colonies, on Sabouraud's agar.

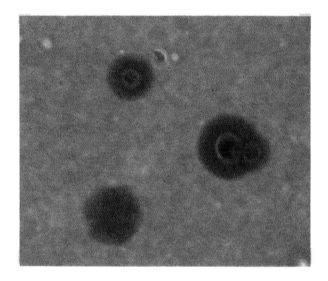

Fig. IV.30. Cryptococcus neoformans. An india ink preparation from a CSF illustrating the large gelatinous capsule which surrounds the organism. The cytoplasmic structure of the cell can be seen, as well as one organism in the budding stage. × 1560.

Chapter 45
Cryptococcosis

Cryptococcosis is an uncommon infection with a world wide distribution. The fungus is found widely in nature although pigeon droppings and nests are generally named as the source of infection. This occurs primarily via the respiratory tract, but direct tissue involvement is also seen. Minimal histological reaction is the rule. The infection is a true blastomycosis as the organism appears in tissues as a budding fungus.

The most severe form of the disease involves the central nervous system and here the leucocyte count from the CSF may be normal or somewhat raised with lymphocytes predominating. The appearance of the CSF is unrewarding, but a pellicle may form. The laboratory findings thus resemble tuberculous meningitis so the causative organism must be demonstrated.

Microscopic examination with the light reduced shows the yeasts but their capsules are not always readily apparent and they may be confused with lymphocytes. India ink preparations show the characteristic morphology of a single yeast 5–20 μ in diameter which may be budding, but in either instance it is surrounded by a wide, refractile, gelatinous capsule which is diagnostic (Fig. IV.30).

Attempts to follow treatment by performing cell counts are usually unsuccessful. Culture is effected at 37°C or room temperature on BA, Sabouraud's or MA plus gentamicin but *not* cycloheximide as the organism is sensitive to this drug. The organisms grow slowly and present as

Fig. IV.31. Undersurface of Cryptococcus neoformans. Note that the surface appearance at 48 hours is similar to *Candida albicans* (Fig. IV.29). The undersurface of cryptococcus is beige in colour, not white.

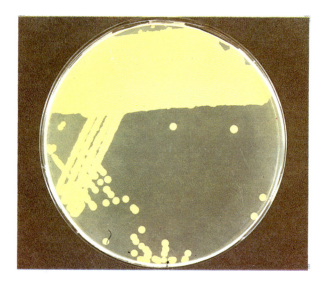

yellowish, mucoid colonies (Fig. IV.31). At this stage no capsule can be demonstrated in microscopic preparations.

Animal inoculation in the mouse can be used to confirm the disease.

Chapter 46
Histoplasmosis (Histoplasma capsulatum)

Histoplasmosis is a primary acute benign pulmonary disease presenting rarely as a progressive, chronic, malignant disease which is caused by *Histoplasma capsulatum*. The disease affects the lungs, bones, skin and mucous membranes.

H. capsulatum differs from all other human pathogenic fungi in that it is primarily a parasite of the reticulo-endothelial system.

The fungus is small with a yeast-like intracellular phase in the tissues of man and a typical mould-like filamentous phase when cultured on Sabouraud's medium at room temperature.

Fresh and unstained clinical specimens are inadequate to demonstrate the fungus, which is best shown in blood or impression smears stained with either Wright's or Giemsa stain.

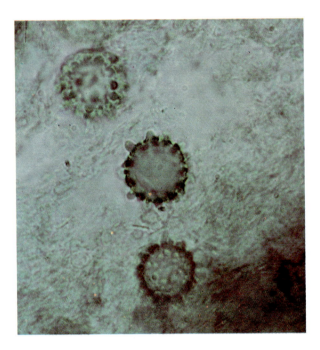

Fig. IV.32. Histoplasma capsulatum.
Lactophenol blue preparation from
Sabouraud's agar shows the typical large
thick walled tubulate chlamydospores
8–14 μ in diameter. × 4342.

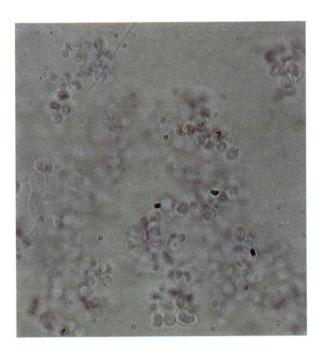

Fig. IV.33. Histoplasma capsulatum.
Lactophenol blue preparation from
glucose cysteine blood agar shows the
characteristic small yeast-like structures,
2 μ × 3 μ in size. × 4342.

The fungus grows from fasting gastric washings or sputum heavily inoculated onto Sabouraud's or brain-heart infusion blood agar with added gentamicin or cycloheximide. The fungus forms white cottony colonies with aerial mycelia which turn buff or brown at room temperature. Colonies resembling *S. albus* are not uncommon. Lactophenol blue preparation of these colonies show the tubulate chlamydospores (Fig. IV.32).

Growth at 37°C on glucose cysteine blood agar gives the parasitic form of the organism. Lactophenol blue preparation of these colonies show the yeast-phase (Fig. IV.33).

All laboratory animals are susceptible regardless of route of inoculation. Extreme care must be taken in the handling of infected animals.

Fig. IV.34. Aspergillus fumigatus.
Spore head. × 2909.

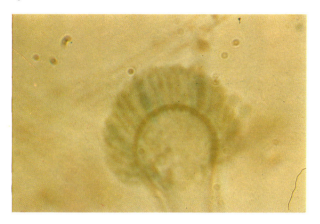

Fig. IV.35. Aspergillus fumigatus.
Broken hyphal elements. × 1336.

Chapter 47
Aspergillosis (Aspergillus Species)

Aspergillus spp. are the most common and troublesome of fungal contaminants in the laboratory. They are found world-wide. Pathogenic members can cause granulomatous lesions of the skin, ears, sinuses, bronchii, lungs and other organs. Infection commonly occurs in patients with lowered host resistance from whatever cause, but healthy individuals are often involved without obvious disease.

Aspergillus fumigatus and *A. niger* are the most common pathogens. *A. clavatus*, *A. flavus* and *A. versicola* are less common causes of disease, and other members of the species are rarely pathogenic.

A proper specimen of sputum pressed onto a slide to make a thin film shows small casts or plugs composed of spore heads embedded in a mycelium (Fig. IV.34), or else broken fragments of hyphae (Fig. IV.35).

Culture on Sabouraud's medium at room temperature leads to a rapidly growing white filamentous colony which quickly turns green to dark green as spores are produced, see Fig. IV.36 (Surface), Fig. IV.37 (Underside).

All species of aspergillus show conidiophores expanding into large terminal vesicles. These surfaces are covered by sterigmata bearing long chains of spores (Fig. IV.38).

For species identification refer to Raper and Fennell, 1965.*

* Raper, K. B. & Fennell, D. (1965) *The Genus Aspergillus.* Williams and Wilkins and Co., Baltimore, pp. 82–126.

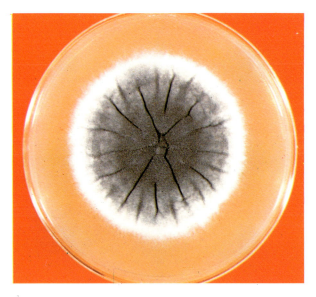

Fig. IV.36. Aspergillus fumigatus
(Surface). Rapidly growing colony. A
convoluted fold forms the central papilla
from which emerge rays of long, slender,
deep grooves touching right up to the
submerged mycelial fringed periphery.
The thallus is greyish green, covered all
over with short aerial mycelial growth.
The fringed edge is of a whitish green.

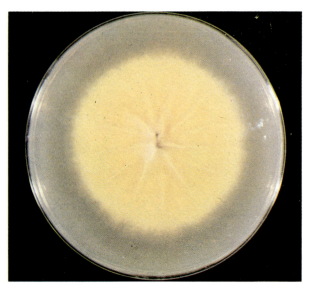

Fig. IV.37. Aspergillus fumigatus
(Underside). The fawn yellow colony
gives the impression of rows of slightly
winding ridges cutting symmetrically all
over the thallus.

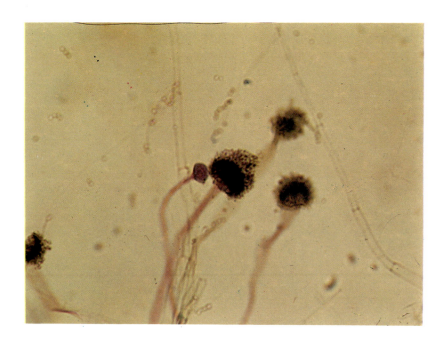

Fig. IV.38. Aspergillus fumigatus.
Growth on Sabouraud's agar for 7 days
shows the septate mycelium in a modified
Riddle slide culture preparation. The
typical conidiophore 2–8 μ wide, expands
into a dome-shaped vesicle 25 μ in
diameter. × 1336.

SECTION V
ANTIBIOTIC
SENSITIVITY
TESTS

Introduction

The *in vitro* testing of antibiotics is the normal way of assessing whether or not a particular organism is sensitive to specific antibacterial agents. At the very best it can only indicate treatment, because the mere fact that a micro-organism *appears* sensitive to one or more anti-biotics on testing in the laboratory is no real guide to the ultimate result achieved in the patient. Although the correct antibiotic may be chosen for a specific infecting organism this takes no heed of the clinical situation where collections of pus requiring surgical drainage, or the concomitant use of immunosuppressive drugs may alter the patient's response even to correct anti-biotic therapy. In brief, *in vitro* testing methods can only be considered, at best, a guide to medical treatment—other factors, e.g. surgical intervention, need to be considered separately but at the same time.

Measures for assessing *in vitro* sensitivity or susceptibility of an infecting organism to certain antimicrobials vary from the most simple to very difficult tests as the Chapters which follow show. In some instances, e.g. the W.H.O. method, it is possible not only to determine sensitivity but also the M.I.C. (Minimum Inhibitory Concentration) of a particular organism at the same time.

The method chosen will vary from laboratory to laboratory dependent on the work-load, finance, etc. But in small laboratories performing such tests only occasionally, simple methods of determining sensitivity will probably be pre- ferred. In a large hospital the bias will obviously be towards one of the more refined (but expensive) methods.

It has been my practise for some years to *test* all available antibiotics, but *report* only the bactericidal ones. There is some merit in this suggestion as it serves to guide the clinician in his treatment of a particular infection. In hospitals, the reporting of *bactericidal* antibiotics *alone* is probably a good thing, but for patients from a General Practice, it is more important that the doctor knows which bacteriostatic antibiotics are useful, as many of the bactericidal drugs are not capable of being used in a General Practice (domiciliary) situation.

Chapter 48
Simple Tests of Sensitivity

(i) Paper Disc Technique

DISCS

This is probably the most popular and simple test used in the hospital diagnostic laboratory. It involves the antibiotic being incorporated in the paper disc. The standard of paper must be such that it has no effect on the organism under test. The concentration of the antibiotic must be chosen with great care so that it will correspond with the results achieved *in vivo*. Today it is possible to obtain discs commercially at the recommended concentration. The results are obtained by the diffusion of the antibiotic into the media causing inhibition of growth.

The conditions of storage of the discs are most important, they should be stored at $-20°C$ or below, and the vials should contain a desiccant. They should be allowed to reach room temperature before being opened, thus avoiding condensation.

The discs normally used for single disc sensitivity testing are penicillin (2 u.), and for the antistaphylococcal penicillins, methicillin (10 μg), cloxacillin (5 μg), perhaps to be replaced by flucloxacillin (5 μg). Broad spectrum penicillins are ampicillin (10 μg), but for urinary tract infections (25 μg) is used. This drug may be replaced by amoxycillin (10 μg). Antipseudomonas penicillins are carbenicillin (100 μg) but perhaps ticarcillin at half the level will be the future drug tested. All these discs are supplied

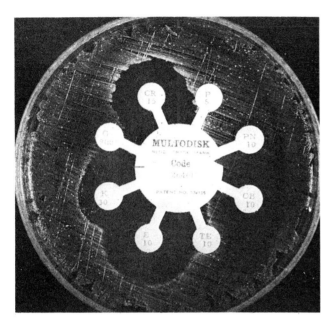

Fig. V.1. Multodisc sensitivity of a S. aureus. Zones of sensitivity to: CR = cephaloridine, K = kanamycin, E = erythromycin. No zone, resistance to: P = penicillin, PN = ampicillin, CB = methicillin, TE = tetracycline and G = sulphonamide.

free of charge by Beecham Research Laboratories. Dicloxacillin (10 μg) is used in the U.S.A. in place of cloxacillin and flucloxacillin. Roussel Laboratories supply gentamicin (10 μg) and framycetin (100 μg) and Schering also give gentamicin. Glaxo Laboratories supply cephaloridine (25 μg) and cephalexin (30 μg) likewise Lederle (Cyanamid) give laboratories minocycline discs (5 μg). An erythromycin disc (10 μg) should also be used for systemic infections, and nitrofurantoin (200 μg) and naladixic acid (30 μg) for urinary tract infections. Sulbenicillin and propyl- and indanyl-penicillin are new drugs for the treatment of pseudomonas infections but are not in general use. Lilly Industries supply cephalothin (30 μg) and

cefazolin (30 μg) discs on request.

A paper to be given soon shows that cephaloridine is the best single familial antibiotic for determining sensitivity of the cephalosporins, whereas dicloxacillin is the best familial member of the isoxazolyl penicllins followed by flucloxacillin.

As well as single commercial discs being available multiple antibiotics can be placed on either a tip, 'Multodisc', or in a ring, 'Mastring', so that up to eight antibiotics can be tested in the one operation—thus making sensitivity testing easier (see Fig. V.1). Another aid to speed is by the use of a dispenser for the single discs which are loaded in cartridges.

Each batch of discs must be tested daily for their efficiency using *S. aureus* Oxford (ATCC

6571), *E. coli* (NCTC 10418) and *P. aeruginosa* (NCTC 1062) as the control organisms.

A method of determining precise sensitivity or resistance using Multodiscs with stringent controls over media, inoculum size, etc., has recently been described.[*]

MEDIA

Many types of media are available for antibiotic sensitivity testing, e.g. Mueller-Hinton agar (B.B.L., Oxoid, Difco), Wellcotest Agar (Wellcome), Oxoid DST agar, but there are a number of alternative commercial preparations available. When selecting media for antibiotic sensitivity testing, various factors need to be taken into consideration, viz. the pH of the agar should be between 7.2–7.4, as many antibiotics are affected by changes in pH, e.g. the aminoglycosides are much more active in an alkaline medium, thus giving a false result if an alkaline medium is used. So, organisms should not be incubated in an atmosphere of CO_2 as this will establish acid conditions, again giving false results. An exception here is when testing sensitivity of the *Neisseria*.

The presence of ions in the medium also has an effect, e.g. the presence of magnesium ion affects the tetracyclines, giving false negative results.

When the media is poured it should be poured on completely level benches to achieve even dis-

[*] Bell, S. M. (1975) 'The CDS Disc Method of Antibiotic Sensitivity Testing (Calibrated Dichotomous Sensitivity Test).' *Pathology*, Vol. 7, No. 4, Suppl.

tribution of the media on the entire plate, i.e. depth should be kept constant, at about 4 mm.

INOCULUM SIZE

This is very important; ideally an overnight broth culture should be used (or a heavily inoculated 2 hour broth culture) and flooded onto the surface of the agar plates, which are not predried. If a 'rapid' antibiogram is required, as often it is in a hospital laboratory 2–5 similar colonies are 'picked off' into broth, flooded as above, discs applied and then allowed to equilibrate at room temperature for $\frac{1}{2}$–1 hour; this result may be readable after 6 hours incubation at 37°C. The ideal inoculum size is that which gives confluent but not dense growth. To achieve this

Staphylococci and *Enterococci* require 10^{-3} organisms/ml, while Gram negative organisms require 10^{-4} organisms/ml.

END-POINT

The obvious end-point is where there is a sudden reduction in growth, which is clear to most observers. The only exceptions are the sulphonamides and the combination of sulphamethoxazole and trimethoprim (which probably should be tested separately, i.e. do not use a single 'combined' disc).

(ii) Incorporation of the Antibiotic in the Media

This method is used in some laboratories and

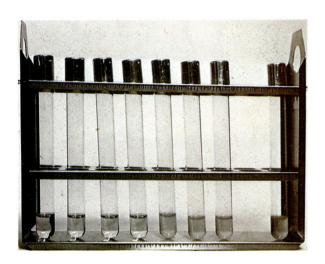

Fig. V.2. Broth dilution technique.
Growth has been inhibited by the antibiotic in the first four tubes; the fourth tube is therefore the Minimum Inhibitory Concentration of the antibiotic as growth has occurred in the last three tubes. It has also occurred in the control tube on the extreme right.

involves the incorporation of an antibiotic at two strengths in two plates. One plate has a high level of antibiotic which if the organism grows will be classed as 'resistant', and the other plate has a much lower level of antibiotic which if the organisms grow can be classed as 'sensitive'. This method allows a control plate with no antibiotic to be added if the plates are inoculated with a replica-plating technique. This technique allows several organisms to be tested against the same antibiotic at the same time.

(iii)   Broth Dilution Tests

In this test doubling dilutions of the antibiotic are necessary. A more sensitive method employs an arithmetic means of dilution of the antibiotic,

but is seldom used. In fact, both are too time-consuming for general use. The result is obtained by inspecting the tubes for growth and the last tube showing complete inhibition of growth is taken as the Minimum Inhibitory Concentration (M.I.C.) of the drug (Fig. V.2). This test is also dependent upon inoculum size, e.g. with car-benicillin the inoculum size should not exceed 10^3 organisms/ml otherwise a falsely high M.I.C. will result. The tubes are normally examined after overnight incubation, i.e. 18 hr at 35–37°C.

(iv)   Gradient Plate Technique

This method has very little use in a routine laboratory, and is mainly used as a screening technique for resistant mutant strains in a bac-

Fig. V.4. Oxford-cup assay method.
Various concentrations of the antibiotic have been added to each cup after they have been placed on a seeded agar plate.

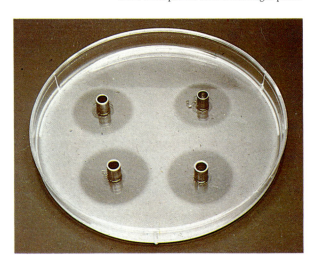

Fig. V.3. Gradient plate technique.
The antibiotic is incorporated in the bottom gradient layer of the plate, and the organism is then added to the surface agar.

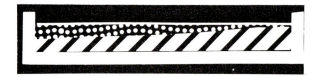

terial population. The agar has the antibiotic incorporated in it and has a gradient of agar slope, thus also of the antibiotic. The organism population under test is then flooded across the surface of the layered agar and then organisms which are resistant will grow up to a certain level of the plate and no further (see Fig. V.3).

(v)   Well Diffusion Technique

This method involves the use of 'punched-out' holes in the agar and the appropriate concentration of antibiotic is added to each hole of a plate previously seeded with the test organism. Again this is a test of diffusion of the antibiotic.

(vi)   Oxford-Cup Assay Method

Again the method is a diffusion test, the agar plate is previously seeded with the test organism and the appropriate concentration of the antibiotic is added to each cup (see Fig. V.4).

(vii)   Direct Sensitivity

The swab is directly swabbed on the Mueller-Hinton plate and is processed as above in Chapter 48. If the culture is mixed, the common antibiotic shows a zone of inhibition—this provides a rapid guide to chemotherapy. Final testing of the individual organisms *must* be repeated the following day to obtain an individual antibiogram for each organism.

Fig. V.5. Regression line. A regression line has been determined for an antibiotic using many test strains of the same organism. From this line the M.I.C. of the organism under test can then be directly obtained by measuring the diameter of the zone of inhibition.

Fig. V.6. W.H.O. method. Zones of inhibition are measured with calipers and the M.I.C. and therefore sensitivity or resistance are determined from the appropriate regression line.

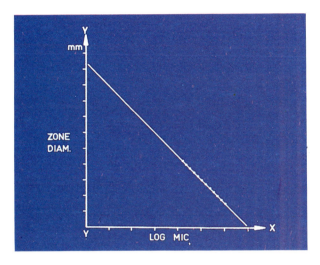

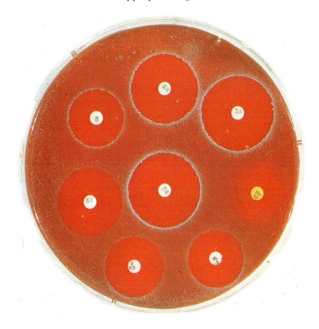

Chapter 49
W.H.O. Method

This method is based on the Report of an International Collaborative Study by Ericsson and Sherris★ (1971). It is based on the disc diffusion technique, and the fact that there is a linear relationship between the zonal inhibition diameter and the log of the M.I.C. of the organism, under standard conditions.

Discs

Each disc is impregnated with a prescribed concentration of antibiotic and stored under the conditions mentioned in Chapter 48. The

★ Ericsson, H. M. & Sherris, J. C. Antibiotic Sensitivity Testing, Report of an International Collaborative Study. *Acta path. microbiol. scand., Sect. B. Suppl.* No. 217.

amount of antibiotic in each disc is determined so that the log of the M.I.C. bears a direct relationship to the zonal diameter of inhibition when measured by a pair of calipers. This means that for a particular antibiotic, the level which can be achieved in the blood of the patient and the M.I.C. of the organism can both be derived from the regression curve. See Figs. V.5 and V.6.

Media

Standard batches of media are used and Mueller-Hinton agar is the medium of choice, with added 5 per cent defibrinated sheep red blood cells, and this is poured into 150 mm diameter Petri dishes. Each plate contains 65 ml of agar which

Fig. V.7. Kirby-Bauer method. The organism under test is classed as 'Susceptible' to the antibiotic in the disc on the left, 'Intermediate' to the centre disc, and 'Resistant' to the one on the right. The results are determined from previous experience with diameters of zonal inhibition for the particular antibiotic under test for the appropriate organism.

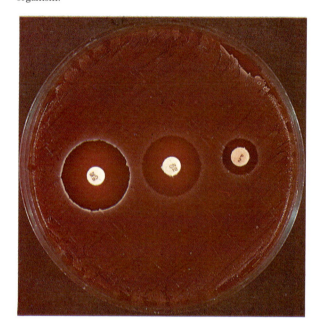

Chapter 50
Kirby-Bauer Method

gives a depth of 4 mm per plate. For each batch of media the regression curve needs to be constructed for each antibiotic.

Inoculum

Five ml of an appropriate diluted culture are flooded over the agar plate, allowed to circulate evenly over the entire plate and then the excess is pipetted off and discarded.

After incubation the zonal diameter of inhibition is recorded in mm using a pair of calipers and then the organism is recorded as sensitive or resistant by referring to the linear curve.

. After trying this method it is not difficult to incorporate in the diagnostic laboratory.

This method is also a single disc method, as described by Bauer, *et al.*★ (1966); they use a standard set of high antibiotic concentrations and dependent on the inhibition zonal diameter the organisms are classed as 'Resistant', 'Intermediate' and 'Susceptible' (see Fig. V.7).

The inoculum is swabbed onto the surface of a Mueller-Hinton agar plate 6 mm deep by the use of a cotton wool swab, and the surplus inoculum is removed by rotating the swab against the side of the plate before use. After overnight incubation the zonal diameter is measured, the end-point being taken as the com-

★ Bauer, A. W., Kirby, W. M. M., Sherris, J. C. & Turck, M. (1966) Antibiotic Susceptibility Testing by a Standardized Single Disk Method. *Amer. J. clin. Path.*, **45**, 493.

Chapter 51
Association of Clinical Pathologists
(Stokes' Method)

plete inhibition of growth (except of sulphona-mides). The results are then read off from the chart which is provided in the paper mentioned above. It is, however, not very satisfactory for slow-growing organisms, e.g. *Neisseria gonor-rhoeae*. To obtain accurate results this method has to be performed with great care.

Once again the method involves the disc dif-fusion of the antibiotic on a suitable agar. The authors recommend the use of specially stan-dardized media to which is added 5 per cent lysed horse blood. The media is poured on a flat surface to a depth of 3–4 mm. The inocu-lum used is that which 'gives dense but not confluent growth' which is evenly distributed over the plate.* Dry swabs are used to inoculate the plate from a loop full of an overnight broth culture or suspension. The discs are placed on the agar and then incubated immediately. The results are read as 'Sensitive', 'Moderately

* Stokes, E. J. & Waterworth, P. M. (1972) Antibiotic Sensitivity Tests by Diffusion Methods. *Association of Clinical Pathologists, Broadsheet* 55.

Fig. V.8. Stokes method. The control organism is cultured onto the top and bottom thirds of the plate, and the organism under test is plated in the centre. It can be seen that the test organism is sensitive to the antibiotic on the top left, and bottom left and right discs, but is resistant to the top right-hand disc.

Fig. V.9. Stokes' method. In this test the organism is only sensitive to the antibiotic on the top left-hand disc.

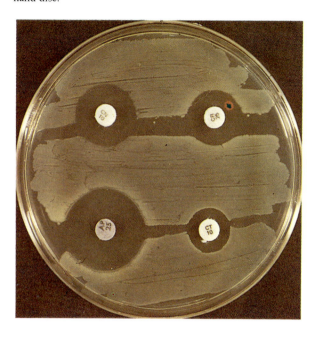

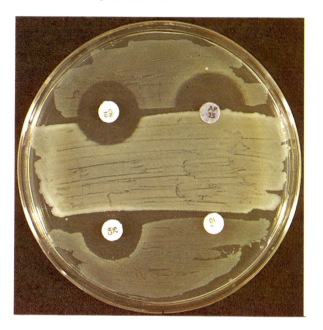

sensitive', and 'Resistant'.

A second method is recommended which incorporates a control culture on either side of the test organism which is inoculated as a band across the centre of the plate (see Fig. V.8 and V.9).

SECTION VI
PARASITOLOGY

Introduction

Although parasitology is a separate discipline distinct from bacteriology, virology, and mycology, it is usually an integral part of the microbiology laboratory. Accurate differential diagnosis is essential to all laboratory disciplines but in parasitology the familiarity of technicians and other professional laboratory personnel in the isolation and recognition of parasitic organisms usually is not well mastered particularly in developed countries where experience with such organisms is infrequent. This shortcoming may be particularly distressing in those countries which have government personnel and their families stationed in numerous tropical and subtropical areas of the world. Also with the advent of jet travel and tourism, large numbers of travellers may be exposed to disease agents with which they are completely unfamiliar regarding prophylactic procedures and clinical symptoms.

In some cases it is possible to accurately identify a parasite from one submitted specimen but this usually is not the case. A concerted effort should, therefore, be made to collect diagnostic specimens in a specified orderly program from the patient. For example, confusion in the accurate diagnosis of malaria has occurred because some medical personnel mistakenly think that a blood smear taken from the patient during a temperature spike is adequate for differential diagnosis. Malarial parasites of all species, however, appear very similar at this point. Instead, blood should be taken at first presentation of the patient and at 6 hour intervals until species differentiation can definitely be established.

Another example which emphasizes the importance of multiple specimen examination is amoebiasis. Cysts and trophozoites of *Entamoeba histolytica* often appear in stool specimens in 'showers', that is, one stool may contain many amoebae while the next stool passed may contain few or no parasites at all.

Most common human parasites are identified directly from faeces or blood, although urine, sputum, and tissue fluids and biopsies occasionally contain organisms. Standard operating procedures should be established for the collection, processing and reporting of results for all of these types of specimens. Consult the appropriate textbooks for details of these procedures.

1 Collection and Treatment of Blood

A. MALARIA

Microscope slides should be washed in warm soapy water, rinsed in ethanol and wiped with a lintless cloth before use. A thick and a thin smear should be made on each slide. This is accomplished by placing a small drop of fresh blood toward one end of a horizontally positioned slide and with the edge of another slide held at a 30° angle making a smooth one-cell thick smear by pulling the drop of blood toward the centre of the slide. On the other end of the slide, a slightly larger drop of blood should be placed. This drop should be circularly spread out to a diameter of 20 mm using the corner of another slide. Both films must be allowed to dry thoroughly whilst kept free from dust, insects, and abrasive materials. Some people prefer not to place a thick and a thin smear on the same slide. This method, however, may lead to separation or mixing of blood smears in the laboratory unless slides are carefully labelled. In either case, slides should be labelled as soon as smears are made as to patient's name, date and time.

The best malaria stain is Giemsa's. First, the thin smear must be fixed by dipping in absolute methanol for a few seconds. Then both thick and thin smears are stained for 60 min in a

1 : 50 dilution of Giemsa pH 7.2 after which the slide should be rinsed thoroughly with Giemsa buffer. Giemsa stain should be used within two hours after the 1 : 50 working dilution is made up. Dried slides may be observed with oil immersion either with or without coverslips. Other malaria stains include: Wright's, Leishman's, J.S.B. and Field's stain.

B. FLAGELLATES

Slides for microscopic diagnosis of trypanosomes should be prepared and stained in a manner identical to those techniques described above for malaria.

Differential diagnosis of the African trypanosomes (*Trypanosoma rhodesiense* and *T. gambiense*) on a morphological basis is impossible so emphasis should be placed on the detection of organisms and the probable geographic source of infection. In cases of suspected African trypanosomiasis it is best to examine not only the blood but also exudate and any enlarged lymph nodes and cerebrospinal fluid as well since organisms usually are absent from peripheral blood in advanced disease. The detection of organisms in one or more of these locations will aid the physician in prognosis and selection of an appropriate treatment schedule. Both African trypanosome species may be cultured in Weinman's medium.

American trypanosomiasis (*T. cruzi*) is characterized by an initial acute stage when organisms are present in peripheral blood. In the subsequent chronic stage, however, trypanosomes usually are not present in blood except during febrile paroxysms. In this case it may be advisable to employ xenodiagnosis (feeding of uninfected triatomid bugs on the patient) to detect active cases. *T. cruzi* may be cultured in Novy, MacNeal and Nicolle's (NNN) medium.

C. FILARIASIS

In suspected cases of filariasis, three procedures should be performed routinely for the detection and subsequent diagnosis of nematodes whose microfilarial stage usually is found in the peripheral blood. These are the wet smear, the thick smear, and the Knott's techniques, all of which can be done using a total of one to two ml of freshly drawn blood. First, a drop or two of blood should be placed on a slide, a coverslip applied, and the sample observed under low power for the presence of living microfilariae which can easily be seen moving in a serpentine fashion through the formed elements of the blood. A Knott's procedure also should be performed to detect active cases where density of microfilariae may be very low. A one ml amount of blood should be thoroughly mixed with 10 ml of two per cent formalin, centrifuged and the sediment examined for microfilariae (immobilized because of formalin fixation). The thick smear, made as in malaria, is used for identification of microfilariae in positive cases. At least two slides should be made, one to be stained with haematoxylin and one with Giemsa to determine nuclear patterns and the presence or absence of a sheath, respectively. If microfilariae are rare, the sediment from a Knott's preparation may be smeared on a slide, allowed to dry and stained as above. Since most filarial infections exhibit a quotidian microfilarial periodicity in the peripheral blood, samples should be taken and examined with the above three methods every 6 hours for at least one entire day.

2 Collection and Treatment of Faeces

Faeces should be collected free of urine, water, or soil in a suitable dry clean container which can be tightly sealed. The labelled specimen (name, time voided, location) if not collected at the laboratory should be taken there as soon as possible after passage. The technician responsible for faecal analysis should conduct a thorough program of analysis as outlined below.

An initial gross macro-examination should be made to characterize the consistency, colour, any unusual odour (for example, foul odour may suggest malabsorption), bulky material (fibres, seeds), abnormal contents (blood, pus, mucous), and macroscopic parasites (round worms, tapeworm proglottids).

Next, two direct slide preparations should be made: (1) saline, and (2) saline with Lugol's iodine. Each is made by mixing about two mg of faeces obtained with the tip of an applicator stick with a few drops of the respective diluent on a microscope slide. A 22 mm² coverslip is applied to each mixture and an immediate and thorough microscopic examination of the complete specimen should be made. If trophozoites of protozoa are present in the faeces they will be seen actively moving in the saline preparation. Protozoan cysts and parasite eggs or motile larvae also may be seen in these samples.

If protozoan cysts or nematode larvae are seen in the saline mount, the Lugol's iodine preparation should be examined. Although protozoan trophozoites are destroyed in this medium, the technician will be able to identify the worm larvae and most protozoan cysts. Helminth eggs are recognizable in either saline or iodine preparations. Although diagnosis of *Entamoeba histolytica* should only be considered as tentative by these methods, all other protozoa usually can be identified using the above preparations.

If protozoan trophozoites of *E. histolytica* cysts are observed in the direct saline preparation, a portion of the faecal specimen should be smeared onto a clean slide and immediately preserved in Schaudinn's fixative or polyvinyl-alcohol (PVA) with subsequent staining with trichrome and/or iron haematoxylin (Noble's short method or Faust's long method).

Regardless of the direct smear results, at least one of the following three concentration methods should be employed for the detection and identification of protozoan cysts and helminth eggs: (1) formalin-ether sedimentation, (2) zinc sulphate flotation, or (3) sugar flotation. The rationale for these procedures is to make use of differences in specific gravity of parasite objects relative to those of the liquid medium and the faecal debris.

The formalin-ether sedimentation technique is particularly useful when dealing with fatty stools since fats and oils are dissolved in the ether layer and thus are removed from the formalin portion where many parasite objects are concentrated. This technique is excellent for separating out the heavier parasite eggs such as those of the trematodes and cestodes. However, this technique does involve more technician time, equipment, and reagents than do the other two techniques. Some workers prefer to use the MIFC (merthiolate-iodine-formaldehyde-concentration) in place of the formalin-ether technique because the former stains all parasite objects a pinkish colour. Otherwise, the two procedures are identical.

The zinc sulphate flotation technique (most common specific gravity used is 1.18) is a rapid method for concentration of most eggs and of protozoan cysts when centrifugation is employed. It is not capable of concentrating worm eggs whose specific gravity is greater than 1.18

(trematodes and most cestodes).

The sugar flotation technique also operates on the flotation theory but has a higher specific gravity (>2.0) than that of zinc sulphate. It is thus useful in the efficient concentration of most parasite objects including eggs of trematodes and cestodes. This technique requires no centrifuge or electrical apparatus so is useful in field operations. However, the method is time-consuming and is quite messy.

Cultivating protozoa for differential diagnosis is not worth the time or money required to perform. If accurate identification cannot be made from initial saline, iodine, and permanent-stained specimens, additional stools should be obtained and the above techniques repeated until a firm diagnosis is made.

Whereas the above techniques provide an opportunity for efficient recovery and accurate identification of parasites in the stool, there sometimes is a need for estimating the intensity of intestinal helminth infections, that is, light, moderate, or heavy. The Stoll dilution egg-count, Beaver's direct smear egg count, and the Kato cleared thick smear techniques should be considered to estimate infection load (see appropriate textbooks for methods).

3 Collection and Treatment of Urine

Urine suspected of containing the flagellate *Trichomonas vaginalis* should be collected in the usual manner and a few drops examined microscopically. If no parasites are seen, the sample should be concentrated by centrifugation and the sediment examined microscopically.

If infection with *Schistosoma haematobium* is suspected, it is very important to collect the last urine passed during an evacuation since the schistosome eggs tend to settle to the bottom of the bladder. The sample should be centrifuged and the sediment examined on a slide.

The presence of any unusual urine contents such as blood or pus also should be noted in addition to any parasites.

4   Collection and Treatment of Sputum

Uncontaminated specimens should be collected in a suitable clean container. A small amount of hydrogen peroxide should be added to the sample to liquefy it for easier examination.

Eggs of the human lung fluke *Paragonimus westermani* often will be macroscopically visible as small reddish flecks in the sputum. These can be picked out of the sample and examined directly on a slide. Even if no flecks are seen, the entire sample should be centrifuged and the sediment examined microscopically.

Fig. VI.1. *Plasmodium* sp. trophozoites (thick smear). Differential diagnosis at this stage is not possible because young trophozoites of all human malarias appear quite similar. All parasites in this figure, however, are in the same stage of development which is suggestive but not diagnostic of *P. falciparum.* × 4342.

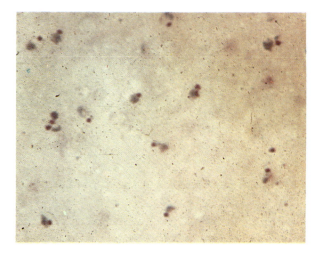

Fig. VI.2. *P. falciparum* trophozoites, ring stage (thin smear). Note the following parasite characteristics which are suggestive of this species: numerous small rings sometimes with double chromatin dots, multiple infection of some host red cells, and parasites sometimes located marginally in the cell. Also note that host red cells are not enlarged. × 4420.

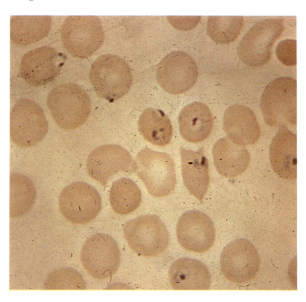

Chapter 52
Malaria

Malaria continues to pose a serious threat to mankind in most tropical and subtropical areas of the world in spite of widespread but often futile efforts to control or eradicate this disease. Medical personnel in developed countries therefore should be aware of the continued possibility of this disease in patients who have a history of travel to areas endemic for malaria and who present with fevers of unknown origin. The consequences of delayed diagnosis of malaria are well exemplified by the record of deaths due to this disease in the United States from 1963 to 1972. In the U.S.A., military and Veterans Administration medical facilities which were continually aware of the threat of malaria experienced a patient death rate which was 24 times less than that of civilian hospitals which were not so accustomed to treating people who had travelled outside the country. In the latter, travel histories of patients frequently were never asked for and thus the possibility of malaria often was not even considered.

Once a postive blood smear has been found, it is extremely important to determine the species of malaria since treatment varies according to the differential diagnosis. Since all human malarial parasites appear similar if obtained during fever paroxysms, it is extremely important to bleed the patient every 6 hours regardless of his symptoms so that parasite development which is characteristic for each species may be observed. It is important to note that all human malarias have

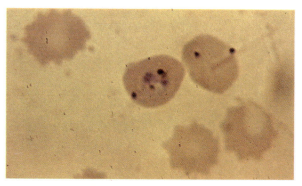

VI.3

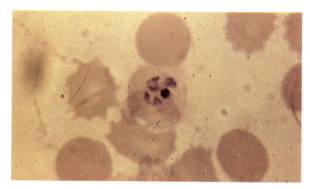

VI.4

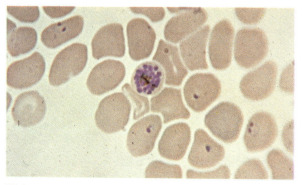

VI.5

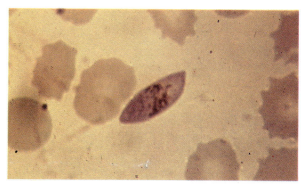

VI.6

Fig. VI.3. *P. falciparum* trophozoites. Note the multiple infections in both red cells in the centre of this figure. The larger parasite in the left red cell is a growing trophozoite showing a compact non-amoeboid shape in contrast to *P. vivax*. Also note that the host red cells are not enlarged and show no Schüffner's dots. The parasite cytoplasm which is normally blue is not visible in this figure because staining was probably done at an acidic pH. × 4420.

Fig. VI.4. *P. falciparum* young schizont. Note the single large clump of pigment and the four chromatin masses inside the normal sized red cell. Again, as in Fig. VI.3, the parasite cytoplasm is not appropriately stained. × 4420.

Fig. VI.5. *P. falciparum* mature schizont. Diagnostic features in this figure include the relatively large number of merozoites (> 12), the normal sized host red cell, and the presence of typical ring stages in other cells. In this figure, typically yellowish-brown pigment is located centrally in the schizont. × 4342.

Fig. VI.6. *P. falciparum* gametocyte. The characteristic cigar shape of this stage is diagnostic for the species. Note the abundant brownish pigment located centrally which obscures the nuclear material. The cytoplasm, normally stained blue, appears reddish in this figure because of the acidic pH of the Giemsa stain used. × 4342.

Fig. VI.7. *Plasmodium* sp. trophozoite ring stage. Although it is virtually impossible to differentiate species at this stage, the rather prominent parasite cytoplasm and the slightly enlarged host red cell in this figure is suggestive of *P. vivax*. × 4420.

Fig. VI.8. *P. vivax* growing trophozoite. Characteristics suggestive of the species at this stage include: the relatively large ring with diffuse greenish-brown pigment and the markedly enlarged host red cell showing Schüffner's dots. × 4420.

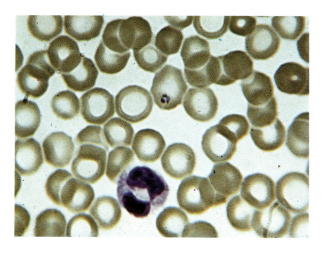

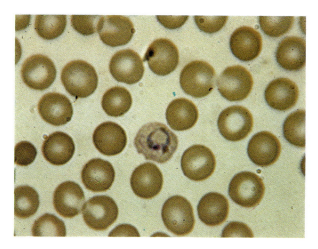

a 48-hour developmental cycle except that of *P. malariae* which is 72 hours. This means there generally is a fever paroxysm every 48 or 72 hours (depending upon the species of plasmodia) due to the bursting of red cells containing mature schizonts which leads to the release of parasite waste products and numerous merozoites. The latter invade new red cells and begin another cyclic growth period which again will result in a subsequent paroxysm.

The photomicrographs in this chapter include pictures from all species of human malaria: *Plasmodium falciparum* (Fig. VI.1–6), *P. vivax* (Fig. VI.7–14), *P. malariae* (Fig. VI.15–17), and *P. ovale* (Fig. VI.18–20). Because of limitations of space all figures except one are of thin blood smears. This omission should not detract from the importance of the thick smear in the detection of very light or mixed malarial infections.

All photomicrographs have been taken from Giemsa stained blood smears. Attention should be paid to the importance of pH of the stain in the demonstration of certain red cell characteristics (for example, Schüffner's dots).

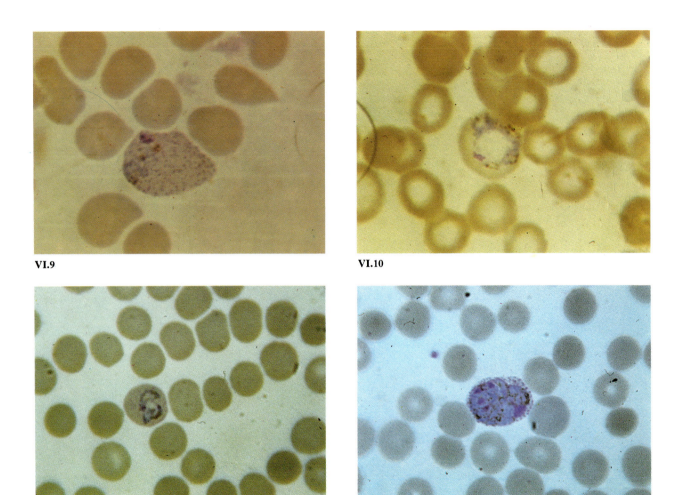

VI.9

VI.10

VI.11

VI.12

Fig. VI.9. *P. vivax* growing trophozoite. Note the characteristic amoeboid shape of the parasite with diffuse greenish-brown pigment and the enlarged host red cell with Schüffner's dots. × 4320.

Fig. VI.10. *P. vivax* mature trophozoite. Note the abundant cytoplasm and the diffuse granular pigment. The enlarged host cell does not exhibit Schüffner's dots in this figure probably because the slide was not stained at an alkaline pH. × 4420.

Fig. VI.11. *P. vivax* young schizont after first nuclear division. Characteristics suggestive of the species at this stage include: amoeboid shape and

diffuse greenish-brown pigment of the parasite, and an enlarged host red cell displaying Schüffner's dots. × 4420.

Fig. VI.12. *P. vivax* immature schizont. This figure shows 5 chromatin masses. Note the characteristically abundant cytoplasm with diffuse greenish-brown pigment and the enlarged host red cell with Schüffner's dots. × 4420.

Fig. VI.13 (top of facing page). *P. vivax* mature schizont. Note the 18 merozoites and the diffuse brownish pigment. The cytoplasm in this stage has largely been divided up among the merozoites. Also note the enlarged host red cell with Schüffner's dots. × 4185.

Fig. VI.14 (top of facing page). *P. vivax* gametocyte. Note the relatively large oval shape of this stage with abundant dark pigment throughout the cytoplasm. This form differs from a mature trophozoite of the same species in that the chromatin is more diffuse and the pigment is more abundant. Again, the host red cell is enlarged but Schüffner's dots are not evident in this figure. × 4420.

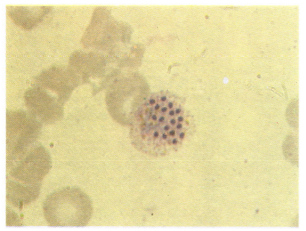

VI.13

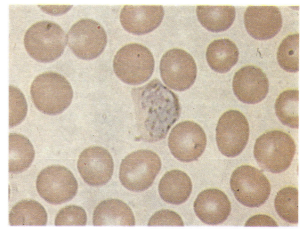

VI.14

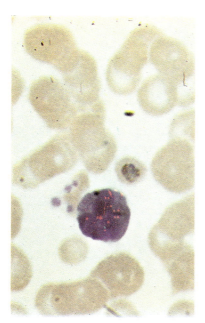

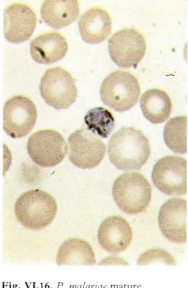

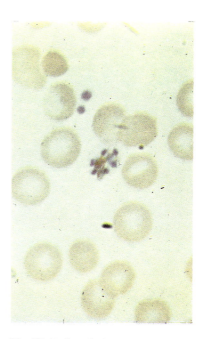

Fig. VI.15. *Plasmodium malariae* growing trophozoite. Note the rather compact cytoplasm with dark brown coarse peripheral pigment. The host red cell is abnormally small. Note the numerous platelets immediately to the left of the neutrophil. These often are mistakenly called young trophozoites of malaria by inexperienced microscopists. However, the distinguishing feature is that no cytoplasm is associated with these reddish bodies. × 4420.

Fig. VI.16. *P. malariae* mature trophozoite. This stage has dense compact cytoplasm and pigment granules which are large, dark, and peripherally arranged. The host red cell which is not visible because the parasite completely fills it, demonstrates the characteristically small size for host cells of this malarial species. × 4420.

Fig. VI.17. *P. malariae* mature schizont. Note the 6 merozoites in a rosette formation with a distinct clump of pigment located centrally. This stage practically fills the abnormally small sized host red cell. × 4342.

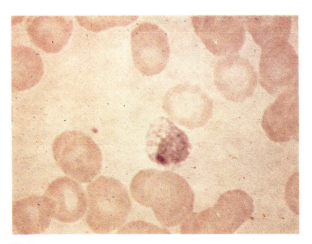

VI.18

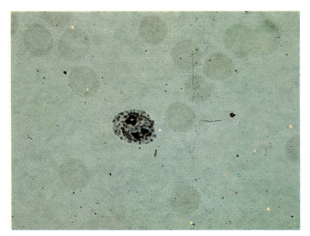

VI.19

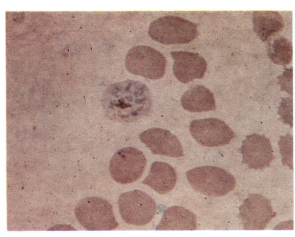

VI.20

Fig. VI.18. *Plasmodium ovale* trophozoite. This stage is rather large and compact in contrast to the amoeboid shape of *P. vivax* and has diffuse inconspicuous pigment. The host red cell is slightly enlarged with Schüffner's dots present but indistinct. × 4420.

Fig. VI.19. *P. ovale* immature schizont with 3 chromatin masses. Note the typically rounded parasite inside the enlarged oval shaped host red cell with distinct Schüffner's dots. × 4342.

Fig. VI.20. *P. ovale* mature schizont. This stage exhibits the typical 8 merozoites in a rosette formation around a central mass of pigment. This differs from *P. malariae* in that the merozoites are larger and the host red cell is oval and slightly enlarged. Schüffner's dots do not show in this figure because staining probably was not done at an alkaline pH. × 4342.

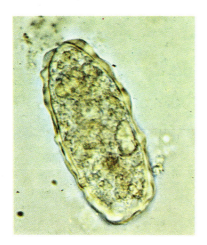

Fig. VI.21. *Ascaris lumbricoides* egg. This specimen is corticated but is unfertilized as evidenced by the yolk completely filling the shell and the oblong shape of the egg. (Unstained) × 1336.

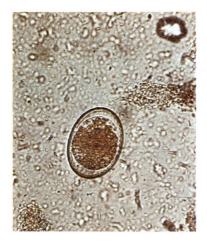

Fig. VI.22. *A. lumbricoides* egg. This fertilized but unsegmented specimen is decorticated and thus may be confused with hookworm. Its shell, however, is much thicker than that of a hookworm egg. This stage also appears somewhat similar to eggs of *S. japonicum* but schistosome eggs are larger and often show the outline of the miracidium inside the egg. (MIF stain.) × 1360.

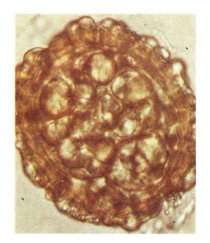

Fig. VI.23 (top right). *A. lumbricoides* egg. Note the pronounced cortication of this fertilized egg, the most commonly seen stage of this parasite. (MIF stain.) × 1336.

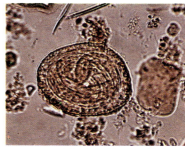

Fig. VI.24. *A. lumbricoides* egg. This decorticated specimen contains a fully developed first stage larva. (MIF stain.) × 1336.

Chapter 53
Nematodes

Roundworm parasites of man inhabit either the tissues (for example, *Wuchereria bancrofti*) or the intestinal tract (for example, hookworm). The most common specimen used for the diagnosis of the latter is faeces since either the worm eggs, larvae, or occasionally the adults will be found there. The pin worm (*Enterobius vermicularis*), however, is most easily detected by the 'Scotch tape technique' since the gravid female migrates to the anus and lays her eggs outside the host's body in the perianal region.

The tissue-inhabiting worms include primarily the filariae; others (for example, the trichina worm) will not be covered in this work. Microfilariae of most filarial worms are found in blood. In some cases, however, the presence of micro-

filariae is not absolutely necessary for a strong presumption of filariasis. For example, many people with advanced elephantiasis never show microfilariae in the peripheral blood although adult worms sometimes may be recovered by lymph node biopsy. Another example is provided by the experience of American troops in the South Pacific during World War II. In spite of hundreds of cases of presumptive filariasis based on various clinical symptoms, almost no patients exhibited microfilaraemia at any time during their illness.

A few filarial parasites, notably *Onchocerca volvulus* and *Dipetalonema streptocerca* have a microfilarial stage which usually is found in the skin, not the blood. Because these parasites will

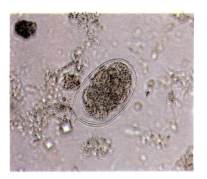
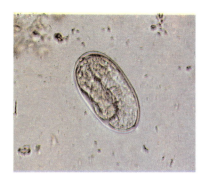

Fig. VI.25. Hookworm sp. egg. This specimen is in the morula stage. Note the very thin wall in comparison with the decorticated *Ascaris* egg. This egg is often mistaken for those of *Trichostrongylus* sp. whose eggs are slightly larger with more pointed ends. × 1360.

Fig. VI.26. Hookworm sp. egg. This specimen contains a fully developed first stage larva. Again note the very thin wall which encloses the larva in an oblong case. (MIF.) × 1360.

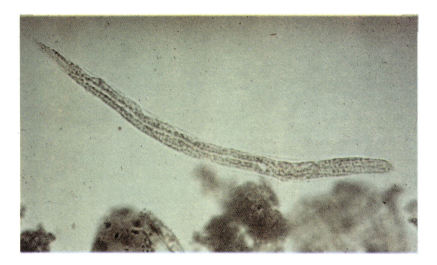

Fig. VI.27. Hookworm sp. rhabditoid larva. This stage shows the following differential characteristics in contrast to that of *Strongyloides stercoralis*. First, a long buccal chamber (not apparent in this figure), second, an inconspicuous genital primordium, and third, a long filiform tail. Staining with Lugol's iodine solution enhances the first characteristic. See Fig. VI.28 for demonstration of a conspicuous genital primordium. × 1336.

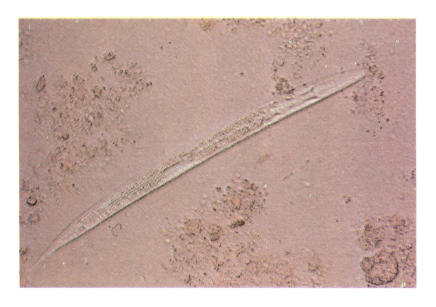

Fig. VI.28. *Strongyloides stercoralis* rhabditoid larva. Compare this stage to hookworm sp. (Fig. VI.27) and note the relatively short buccal chamber, the conspicuous genital primordium (immediately posterior to the midpoint of the worm), and the relatively stubby tail. (MIF stain.) × 1360.

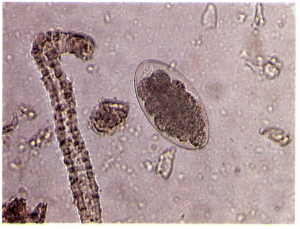

VI.29

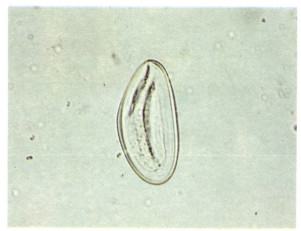

VI.30

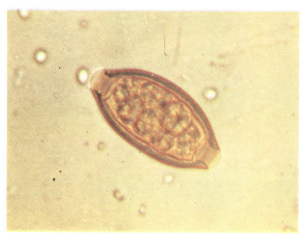

VI.31

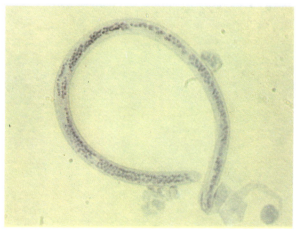

VI.32

not be covered in this atlas, the student is advised to consult a parasitology or tropical medicine text.

Illustrations of the nematodes covered in this work are found in Fig. VI.21–37.

Fig. VI.29. *Trichostrongylus* sp. egg. The thin wall and general shape of this morula stage closely resembles that of hookworm. This egg is slightly larger than that of hookworm, however, and is more pointed, particularly at one end. (Iodine stain.) × 1336.

Fig. VI.30. *Enterobius vermicularis* egg. This photomicrograph shows a typically ovoidal egg which is flattened on one side and convex on the other. Note the enclosed larva. (Unstained.) × 1336.

Fig. VI.31. *Trichuris trichiura* egg. Note the characteristic barrel shape with the bipolar mucoid plugs and the triple-walled shell which easily distinguishes this species. This egg is in the morula stage. (Iodine stain.) × 1291.

Fig. VI.32. *Wuchereria bancrofti* microfilaria. This sheathed first stage larva shows a cephalic space (absence of nuclei at the anterior end) which is equal in length and breadth, a tapered tail with terminal nuclei absent, and well defined body nuclei. (Haematoxylin stain.) × 1336.

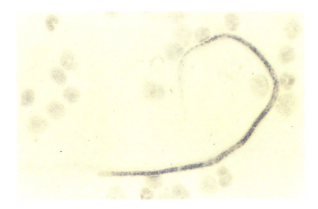

Fig. VI.33. *Brugia malayi* microfilaria. This species may be differentiated from *W. bancrofti* in a number of ways: (1) it is about 20 per cent shorter in length, (2) the cephalic space is twice as long as broad, and (3) the tapered tail contains 2 terminal nuclei. (Haematoxylin stain.) × 1336.

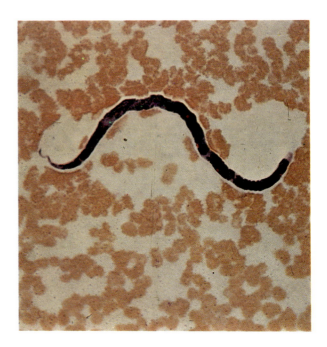

Fig. VI.34. *Loa loa* microfilaria. This species is distinctive from both *W. bancrofti* and *B. malayi* in that its body nuclei are larger and there is a single continuous row of large caudal nuclei which extends to the tail tip. The sheath of this species is difficult to demonstrate and is not visible in this figure. (Giemsa stain.) × 1336.

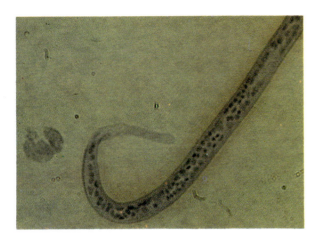

Fig. VI.35. *W. bancrofti* microfilaria. Note that the caudal nuclei do not extend to the tail tip. Also note the sheath which extends beyond the tail. (Haematoxylin stain.) × 3006.

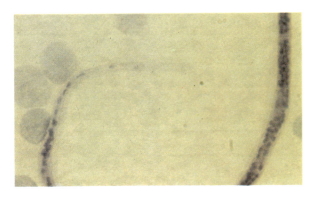

Fig. VI.36. *B. malayi* microfilaria. The tail of this species clearly shows 2 terminal nuclei in the extreme tip. Again note the extension of the sheath beyond the tail. (Haematoxylin stain.) × 3006.

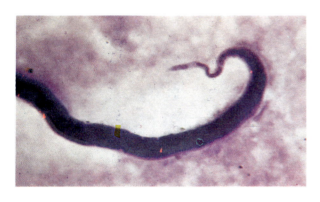

Fig. VI.37. *L. loa* microfilaria. This figure clearly shows a single row of large oblong nuclei extending to the extreme tip of the tail. The sheath is not evident. (Giemsa stain.) × 2925.

Chapter 54
Cestodes

Relatively few species of tapeworms parasitize man. Of those covered in this work, all except one (*Echinococcus granulosus*) inhabit the intestinal tract. Two species of *Taenia* are found in man (*T. saginata* and *T. solium*) but they cannot be differentiated by their eggs. These two species can easily be separated, however, if proglottids are passed by noting their general shape and the number of lateral uterine branches each contains (see appropriate textbooks for details).

E. granulosus would be seen in the laboratory only after an operation was performed on a patient infected with the hydatid cyst of this parasite. This stage is a hollow tumour commonly found growing in the liver that contains 'hydatid sand' which under the microscope appears as

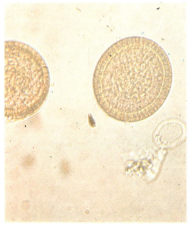

VI.38

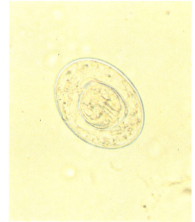

VI.39

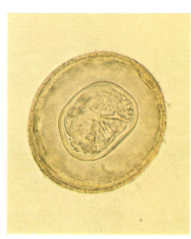

VI.40

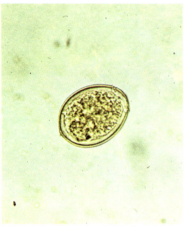

VI.41

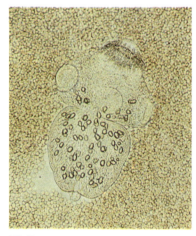

VI.42

hundreds of scoleces as in Fig. VI.42.

Photomicrographs of the more medically important cestode species are illustrated in Fig. VI.38–42.

Fig. VI.38. *Taenia* sp. egg. This photomicrograph shows the characteristic thick-walled, radially striated shell which is spherical in shape. The enclosed onchosphere with its 6 hooks usually can be seen. (MIF stain.) × 1336.

Fig. VI.39. *Hymenolepis nana* egg. The smooth outer shell of this species is nearly spherical and encloses an onchosphere within which can be seen 3 of the 6 hooklets in this focal plane. Note the polar filaments originating from diametrically opposed polar thickenings on the exterior of the onchosphere. These filaments fill up most of the clear space between the onchosphere and the outer shell. (Unstained.) × 1336.

Fig. VI.40. *H. diminuta* egg. This species appears very similar to *H. nana* but may be distinguished by its greater size and larger space between the onchosphere and outer shell with a complete lack of polar filaments. Note that 4 of the 6 onchosphere hooklets are visible in this focal plane. (Unstained.) × 1336.

Fig. VI.41. *Diphyllobothrium latum* egg. This ovoid egg shows a prominent operculum and also a knob (boss) on the opposite (abopercular) end. In contrast to those of the fasciolids, these eggs are smaller and have a larger, more prominent operculum. (Unstained.) × 1336.

Fig. VI.42. *Echinococcus granulosus* scolex. This specimen which originates from the hydatid cyst clearly shows 4 suckers with a rostellum armed with numerous hooklets. (Unstained.) × 129.

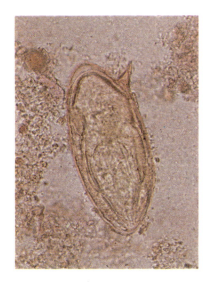 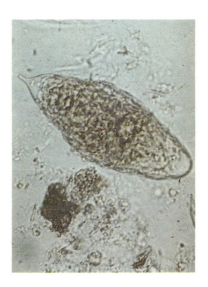 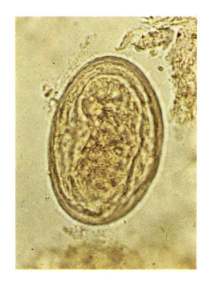

Fig. VI.43. *Schistosoma mansoni* egg. This large egg with the prominent thorn-like lateral spine is easily distinguishable from all other helminth eggs. The fully developed miracidium is clearly visible through the transparent ovoidal shell. (MIF stain.) × 1336.

Fig. VI.44. *S. haematobium* egg. Eggs of this species also are unique from those of all other helminths due to the prominent terminal spine. The miracidium inside the transparent ovoid-shaped shell has deteriorated due to prolonged fixation. (Unstained.) × 1360.

Fig. VI.45. *S. japonicum* egg. Note the distinctly smaller size of this ovoid egg in comparison to that of the other schistosome species. The abbreviated lateral spine, rarely seen because of its small size, is clearly visible at 10 o'clock in this photomicrograph. (Iodine stain.) × 1336.

Chapter 55
Trematodes

The flukes which parasitize man represent a very heterogeneous group as exemplified by the numerous locations where adult worms can be found in the human host. For example, adult schistosomes are located in the blood-vascular system, *Paragonimus* in the lungs, *Clonorchis* and *Fasciola* in the biliary system, and *Metagonimus* in the intestinal tract. Eggs of most trematodes, however, are found in the faeces except for *S. haematobium* (urine) and *P. westermani* (sputum).

Eggs of *C. sinensis* are very difficult to differentiate from a number of other trematodes infecting man (for example, *Opisthorchis*, *Metagonimus*, and *Heterophyes*). Similarly, *Fasciola hepatica* eggs appear very similar to those of *Fasciola gigantica* and *Fasciolopsis buski* (consult appropriate textbooks).

Trematodes illustrated in this text are found in Fig. VI.43–48.

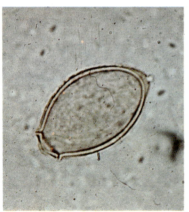

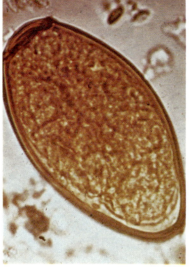
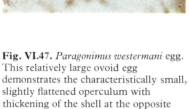
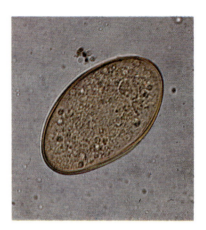

Fig. VI.46. *Clonorchis sinensis* egg. This specimen exhibits the typically pyriform shape, the prominent operculum, and the small knob (boss) at the opposite (abopercular) end. Note the conspicuous shoulders on the shell on either side of the operculum. The outline of the miracidium is visible in this figure. (Unstained.) × 3006.

Fig. VI.47. *Paragonimus westermani* egg. This relatively large ovoid egg demonstrates the characteristically small, slightly flattened operculum with thickening of the shell at the opposite (abopercular) end. (MIF stain.) × 1336.

Fig. VI.48. *Fasciola hepatica* egg. The extremely large size of this oval egg easily differentiates this species from all others except other fasciolids (see Introduction). Note the very small inconspicuous operculum at the top of the figure. (MIF stain.) × 1336.

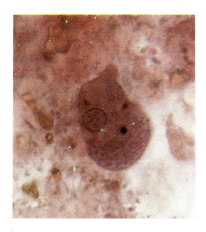

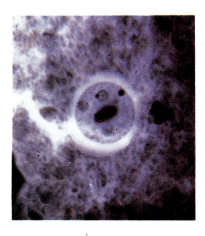

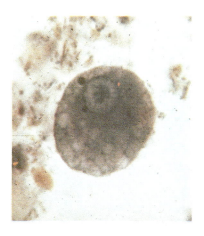

Fig. VI.49. *Entamoeba histolytica* trophozoite. This specimen demonstrates the typically delicate nuclear membrane with the enclosed karyosome (usually centrally located in this species but slightly eccentric in this photomicrograph). Note the dark fragments of several ingested red blood cells in the cytoplasm; also the pseudopod toward the top of the figure. (MIF stain.) ×4420.

Fig. VI.50. *E. histolytica cyst.* This photomicrograph shows 3 of the 4 nuclei with centrally located karyosomes in this focal plane. Also, the single chromatin bar shows the characteristically smooth rounded ends. (Iron haematoxylin stain.) ×4420.

Fig. VI.51. *E. coli* trophozoite. Features which distinguish this species from *E. histolytica* include: (1) the relatively coarse karyosome, (2) the coarse chromatin granules lining the nuclear membrane, (3) the lack of ingested red blood cells in the cytoplasm, and (4) the usual larger body size. (Haematoxylin stain.) ×4420.

Chapter 56
Protozoa

Most protozoa which infect man are found in the intestinal tract, the most pathogenic of which is *Entamoeba histolytica*. Of paramount importance in the laboratory is the accurate detection of this organism which looks much like many other gut protozoa to the inexperienced microscopist. Once this primary objective of determining whether an organism is or is not *E. histolytica* has been achieved, it is of lesser importance to identify the other protozoa since most are not pathogenic to man. The two most commonly committed errors in the diagnosis of *E. histolytica* are: (1) calling this organism *E. coli* or *vice versa*, and (2) mistaking the numerous degenerating white blood cells found in diarrhoea stools (for example, shigellosis) for *E. histolytica* cysts.

Non-intestinal dwelling protozoa pictured in this atlas include the trypanosomes, *Trichomonas vaginalis* and the plasmodia.

Photomicrographs of the major non-malarial protozoa found in man are pictured in Figs. VI.49–67.

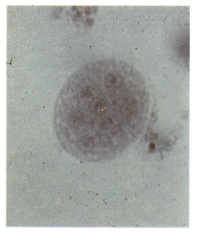

VI.52

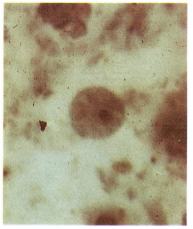

VI.53

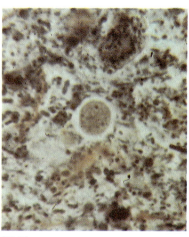

VI.54

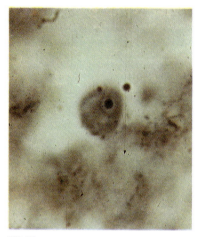

VI.55

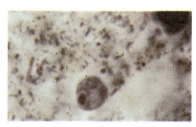

VI.56

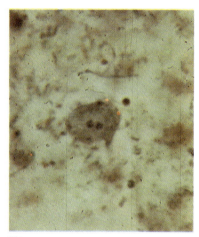

VI.57

trophozoite, however, may be very difficult to differentiate from that of *Iodamoeba bütschlii* (Fig. VI.55). *E. nana* usually has a more centrally located karyosome. (Trichrome stain.) × 4342.

Fig. VI.54. *E. nana* cyst. Although this species generally has 4 nuclei in its cyst stage as does *E. histolytica*, the relatively large nuclear karyosome of *E. nana* distinguish the two species. (Iron haematoxylin stain.) × 4342.

Fig. VI.55. *Iodamoeba bütschlii* trophozoite. This species has highly vacuolated cytoplasm and a very large, dark, usually eccentrically positioned karyosome. The nuclear characteristics clearly distinguish this species from *E. histoly* though differentiation from trophozoites of *E. nana* is often difficult (see Fig. VI.53). (Iron haematoxylin stain.) × 4342.

Fig. VI.56. *I. bütschlii* cyst. Note the large light coloured glycogen vacuole (this will stain brown with iodine) which is present in cysts of this species. In

Fig. VI.52. *E. coli* cyst. Note that 6 of the 8 nuclei are visible in this focal plane. *E. histolytica* cysts seldom contain more than 4 nuclei and generally are smaller than *E. coli*. Although not present in this figure, chromatoidal bars with jagged ends often are present in cysts of this species (as opposed to bars with rounded ends in *E. histolytica*). (Iron haematoxylin stain.) × 4420.

Fig. VI.53. *Endolimax nana* trophozoite. Note the highly vacuolated cytoplasm and the very large dark karyosome with a narrow nuclear clear space (halo effect) surrounding it. The nuclear characteristics serve to distinguish this species from *E. histolytica*. This

this figure, the large karyosome is partially surrounded by the characteristic crescent of dark chromatin granules over its upper edge. (Iron haematoxylin stain.) × 4342.

Fig. VI.57. *Dientamoeba fragilis* trophozoite. The characteristic binucleate structure of this species distinguishes it from trophozoites of all other amoebae. Note the tetrad arrangement of the four chromatin granules in each nucleus. The nuclear membranes are delicate and lack peripheral chromatin. The cyst stage of this species is not known. (Iron haematoxylin stain.) × 4342.

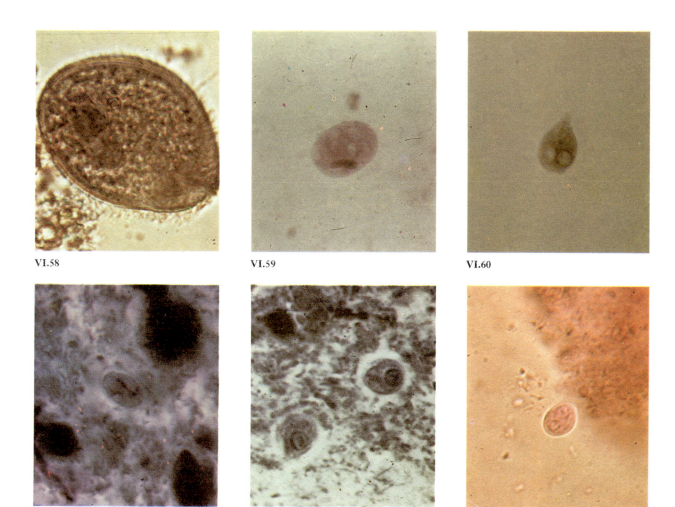

VI.58

VI.59

VI.60

VI.61

VI.62

VI.63

Fig. VI.58. *Balantidium coli* trophozoite. Characteristics of this protozoan, the largest which infects man, include the prominent cytostome at the slightly constricted end, the dark-staining macronucleus, and the cilia. (MIF stain.) × 1336.

Fig. VI.59. *B. coli* cyst. As with the trophozoite of the species, this stage also is characteristically large. Also note the dark-staining macronucleus. (MIF stain.) × 400.

Fig. VI.60. *Giardia lamblia* trophozoite. Note the pear-shaped body with a sharply attenuated posterior end with two subspherical nuclei which together resemble an owl's face. Also note the dark-staining parabasal body immediately posterior to the nuclei. Flagella are not visible in this figure. (Iron haematoxylin stain.) × 4342.

Fig. VI.61. *G. lamblia* cyst. This easily recognized form shows only 1 of the 4 cyst nuclei in this focal plane at 2 o'clock. Also note the curved parabasal body at 8 o'clock and the dark-staining longitudinal axonemes. (Iron haematoxylin stain.) × 4342.

Fig. VI.62. *Chilomastix mesnili* trophozoites. Note the teardrop shape with a single nucleus containing an irregularly shaped karyosome. Also note the darkly stained cytostomal fibrils; however, the flagella do not stain in this preparation. (Iron haematoxylin stain.) × 4342.

Fig. VI.63. *C. mesnili* cyst. This stage generally assumes a pear or lemon shape which clearly identifies this species even when internal structures may not be visible. The nucleus and cytostomal fibrils are visible but indistinct in this figure. (MIF stain.) × 4342.

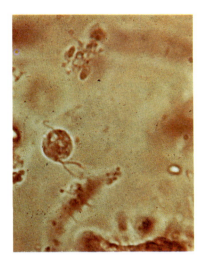

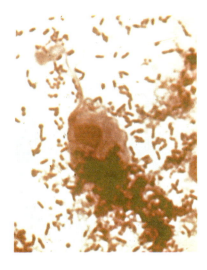

Fig. VI.64 (left). *Trichomonas hominis* trophozoite. Note the distinct flagella in this form; however, the nucleus and axostyle are not visible in this preparation. (MIF stain.) × 4234.

Fig. VI.65. *T. vaginalis* trophozoite. Note the anterior flagella (top), the dark red nucleus, and the undulating membrane (right side) of this urogenital-dwelling flagellate. If urine and faeces become mixed, this species may be differentiated from *T. hominis* by its considerably larger size. (Eosin stain.) × 4234.

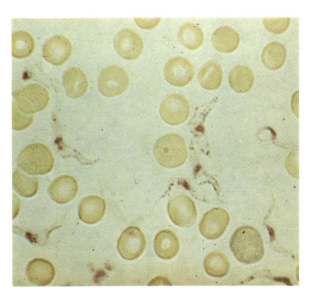

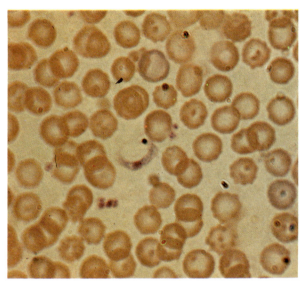

Fig. VI.66. *Trypanosoma* sp. The two species of trypanosomes causing African sleeping sickness (*T. gambiense* and *T. rhodesiense*) are not morphologically distinguishable. Note the large spindle-shaped body with a very small blepharoplast in contrast to that of *T. cruzi* (Fig. VI.67). (Giemsa stain.) × 4290.

Fig. VI.67. *T. cruzi*. This haemoflagellate is found only in the Western world and is easily distinguishable from the African trypanosomes. *T. cruzi* has a relatively small body (often assuming a 'C' shape) which contains a very large blepharoplast. (Giemsa stain.) × 4290.

SECTION VII
VIROLOGY

Introduction

The following types of test are used in the laboratory diagnosis of viral disease:

1　Microscopic examination of clinical or autopsy material for evidence of infection.
2　Isolation and characterization of the infecting virus.
3　Serological determination of recent infection in the patient (see Chapter 64).
4　Identification of viral antigens.

For the diagnosis of most viral diseases, it is neither possible nor necessary to apply each kind of test; the type(s) of test(s) preferred will depend upon the nature and availability of the specimen and on particular characteristics of the virus isolation being attempted. The principal

Table VII.1. Microscopic features of virus-infected cells.

| Virus group | Virus type | Presence of inclusion bodies | | Presence of syncytia |
		Nuclear	*Cytoplasmic*	
Poxvirus	Smallpox	—	Eosinophilic★ (Guarnieri bodies)	
Herpesvirus	Varicella/zoster Herpes simplex	Eosinophilic★	—	+ ★
	Cytomegalovirus	Eosinophilic★	Eosinophilic★	+ ★
Adenovirus	Various types	Basophilic	—	− ‡
Reovirus	Various types	—	Eosinophilic (Perinuclear inclusion)	
Paramyxovirus	Measles	Eosinophilic★	Eosinophilic★	+ ★
	Parainfluenza viruses	—	Eosinophilic	+ ★
Rhabdoviruses	Rabies	—	Eosinophilic★ (Negri bodies)	
Myxoviruses	Various types	Eosinophilic†	Eosinophilic†	
Alpha- and Flaviviruses	Most types	Eosinophilic†	Eosinophilic†	
	Yellow fever	Eosinophilic★ in liver cells (Torres bodies)		
Picornaviruses	Polioviruses Echoviruses Coxsackieviruses	—	—	

★ Commonly used for the diagnosis of infection.
† Occurrence is variable in different hosts.
‡ Focal aggregation of cells without fusion of outer membrane.

laboratory methods used in viral diagnosis will be given in the following chapters and this will be followed by a summary of procedures most applicable to the isolation of viruses of clinical significance.

1 Microscopic Examination of Clinical or Autopsy Specimens

Tests of this kind have been used for many years in India in the diagnosis of rabies or for the differentiation of smallpox and varicella, which in the initial stages of infection are often clinically similar. The test is rapid but applicable only to viruses which induce the formation of well-marked inclusion bodies or syncytia in the cells they infect. Impression smears and scrapings from skin or vesicle fluid are the best sources of material for microscopic examination. Slide preparations are first fixed with Bouin's or Zenker's fluid and then stained with haematoxylin and eosin or May-Grunwald-Giemsa stains. A summary of the principal microscopic features of infection by the various virus groups is given in Table VII.1.

By the application of highly-specific immuno-fluorescence techniques the use of direct microscopy has been extended considerably in recent years and is of particular value where inclusion bodies are either absent or difficult to detect in susceptible cells. In the case of rabies virus infections, an immunofluorescence test has been adopted by the World Health Organization as the standard diagnostic procedure.

There has been an increasing use of electron microscopy for the differential diagnosis of smallpox and other vesicular diseases in recent years, but this technique must still be regarded as beyond the scope of most routine hospital laboratories.

Key to Abbreviations in Virology

EAL	Allantoic cavity of embryonated eggs.
EAM	Amniotic sac of embryonated eggs.
EChor	Chorion of embryonated eggs.
HA	Haemagglutination.
Had	Haemadsorption.
Ham	Human amnion cell cultures.
HEK	Human embryonic kidney cell cultures.
HEF	Human embryonic fibroblast cell cultures (usually a cell strain).
He La	Hetty Lane Line
HEp-2	Human epithelial line no. 2.
IB	Presence of virus-specific inclusion bodies.
ID	Immunodiffusion
IF	Immunofluorescence.
PIC	Primate kidney cell cultures.

Chapter 57
Virus Isolation Procedures

1 Cell Cultures—Preparation

The isolation of most viruses is best accomplished in cell (often mistakenly referred to as 'tissue') cultures. The cell cultures most commonly used are:

(a) Cells of epithelial origin derived from human embryo kidney, human amnion or from primate kidneys, generally those of rhesus or cynomalgous monkeys. After growth, these primary cultures may be used for virus isolation or they may be used after subculture to produce secondary cultures.

(b) Human fibroblast cell strains, which are maintained in the diploid state for approximately fifty subcultures and can be stored in liquid nitrogen and thawed for repropagation as required.

(c) Continuous cell lines of malignant origin which can be subcultured indefinitely and stored in liquid nitrogen under the same conditions as for cell strains.

Primary cell cultures are prepared by dispersing whole organs (for example—kidney, skin) with trypsin, resuspending in growth medium at a suitable cell concentration and inoculating to screw-capped tubes. The cultures are incubated at $37°C$ in a slanting position until growth has occurred. Cultures prepared from cell strains and cell lines are also dispersed with trypsin, but in the presence of a suitable chelating agent such as versene.

Table VII.2. Production of CPE in cell culture by members of the major virus groups.

Virus group	Type of CPE	Time for observations
Picornaviruses	Cells become rounded, refractile and then retract. Complete degeneration of cells results.	3–4 days
Few Picornaviruses e.g. Rhinoviruses Reoviruses	Cells become rounded, refractile then retract. Complete degeneration of cells results.	7–14 days
Some Alphaviruses	,, ,,	3–4 days
Adenoviruses	Focal aggregation, followed by release of cells into medium	1–4 weeks
Most Herpesviruses	Formation of multinucleate syncytia, followed by focal degeneration of cell layer.	3–4 days
Some Herpesviruses Paramyxoviruses	,, ,,	1–4 weeks
Rhabdoviruses Coronaviruses Myxoviruses Some Alphaviruses Some Flaviviruses	Some release of cells into medium, but little overt cell degeneration.	5–7 days
Some Flaviviruses, (including rubella) Arenaviruses	Minimal cell degeneration.	1–4 weeks

The growth medium will vary according to the particular cell type. It usually consists of a synthetic base such as Medium 199, Eagles Basal or Minimal Essential Medium with 5–10 per cent serum (often foetal calf) with other additives such as tryptose phosphate broth, lactalbumin hydrolysate or chick embryo extract being added as required. Sodium bicarbonate (0.15–0.25 per cent w/v) is included to maintain the cells at a pH suitable for cell and virus growth.

2 Use of Cell Cultures for Virus Isolation

Cultures prepared in screw-capped tubes should be used a day before cell confluence has been attained. Specimens, whose collection is described in Chapter 19, are inoculated in 0.1 ml amounts and the tubes transferred to slowly rotating roller-drums held in a 37°C warm room. For attempted isolations of rhinoviruses, incubation at 30–33°C is necessary.

Tube cultures are examined frequently under a light microscope for evidence of infection and are compared with uninoculated control cultures. The observation period will depend upon the nature of the virus suspected to be present, which is based upon a preliminary clinical assessment of the disease.

Virus growth can usually be recognized by a specific pattern of cell destruction, referred to as

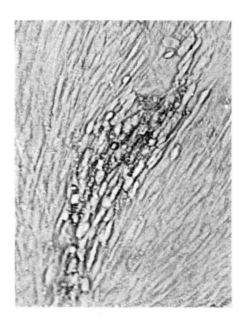

Fig. VII.1. Production of early CPE by cytomegalovirus. Human embryo fibroblast cultures in roller tubes were infected with a preparation of cytomegalovirus. A refractile focus of infected cells can be seen after 8 days.

a cytopathic effect (CPE), which is characteristic for different groups of viruses.

A list of the types of CPE produced by major virus groups and the time taken for each to occur is presented in Table VII.2. An example of the type of CPE produced by cytomegalovirus is given in Fig. VII.1.

CYTOTOXICITY IN SPECIMENS

Some specimens are highly cytotoxic and their destructive effects upon cells in the culture may be confused with a virus-induced CPE. However, with cytoxicity, complete degeneration of the cells occurs within 24 hours whereas at least 2–3 days is usually required for virus-induced

cell degeneration to occur. Cytoxicity may be minimized by removing the medium from the cell culture, adding the inoculum directly to the cell sheet in a small volume and allowing it to act for 1–2 hours at 37°C. The inoculum fluid is then removed by rinsing several times with buffered saline and replaced by a maintenance medium of a lower serum content (1–3 per cent) than that of the original growth medium.

FURTHER DEFINITION OF THE VIRUS PRODUCING A CPE

Full characterization of the virus in cell culture may be achieved serologically by tests of neutralization, complement fixation or immunodiffusion (see Chapter 64).

Chapter 58
Tests for Haemadsorption

Some preliminary information on the nature of the agent may be obtained from observations of the type of CPE produced in cell culture (see Table VII.2), but further definition is described in the following chapters.

Some viruses have the property of attaching to the outer surfaces of red blood cells, causing suspensions of cells to settle rapidly in a characteristic pattern known as haemagglutination. The use of haemagglutination for the diagnosis of infection will be discussed in Chapter 61 describing the use of embryonated eggs.

Many haemagglutinating viruses are released from cells by budding from the outer membrane. Before release, viral haemagglutinating proteins (haemagglutinins) are incorporated in the membrane, allowing the attachment of red blood cells to infected cells.

In order to test for haemadsorption, medium is removed from an infected cell culture and replaced with 0.2 ml of a 0.4 per cent suspension

Fig. VII.2. Haemadsorption in influenza virus—infected monkey kidney cell cultures. Medium from a 3-day infected cell culture was removed and the culture treated with a suspension of 0.4 per cent chicken red blood cells. After 30 minutes, non-attached red cells were removed by rinsing several times with phosphate buffered saline. Specifically adhering red cells can be seen. × 301.

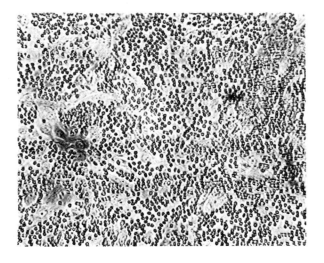

of chicken or guinea pig red cells. The infected culture is held in a slanted position for 30 minutes and then washed several times in buffered saline before examining microscopically. An infected culture showing haemadsorption is shown in Fig. VII.2.

Haemadsorption may be used to detect the presence of myxoviruses, paramyxoviruses and many alpha- and flaviviruses. Diagnosis by this method is rapid and is particularly useful for slow-growing viruses and viruses which produce little CPE.

Chapter 59
Staining for Inclusion Bodies

The formation of inclusion bodies or multinucleate syncytia is pathognomonic of infection by many viruses and the direct examination of infected tissues has been described in the introduction to this section. Infected cell cultures may also be examined for inclusions and syncytia as flat mounted preparations. Preparations of two kinds may be examined:

(i) Cells may be cultured on coverslips in screw-capped tubes and then infected. At a time suitable for examination, the coverslip is fixed, stained and mounted.

(ii) The cell layer from an infected tube culture may be embedded in collodion and then transferred to the surface of a glass slide. The collodion is removed with a suitable solvent and

Fig. VII.3. Inclusion body formation by herpes simplex virus. Coverslip cultures of human fibroblasts were infected with herpes simplex virus. After 3 days, the cultures were fixed, stained and mounted. Arrows indicate the presence of intranuclear inclusion bodies. × 2104.

Fig. VII.4. Formation of multinucleate syncytia by respiratory syncytial virus. Coverslip cultures of HEp-2 cells were fixed, stained and mounted 3 weeks after infection. Two multinucleate syncytia can be seen. × 2104.

Fig. VII.5. Perinuclear inclusion body formation by a reovirus. Cultures of primary cynomalgous monkey kidney cells were prepared on coverslips and infected with a reovirus. Perinuclear inclusion bodies (indicated by arrows) can be seen in the stained preparation after 5 days. × 2104.

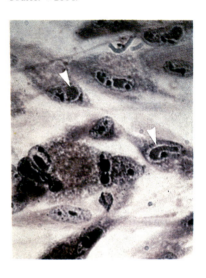

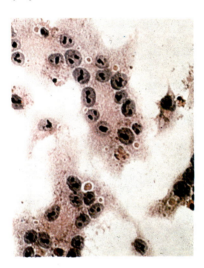

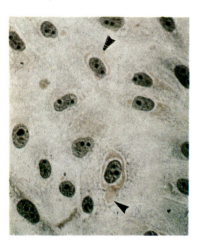

the cells fixed and stained and mounted under a coverslip.

The induction of inclusion bodies and multinucleate syncytia in cells by different viruses is described in Table VII.1. Specific examples of intranuclear and perinuclear inclusions and syncytium formation are shown in Fig. VII.3, Fig. VII.4, Fig. VII.5.

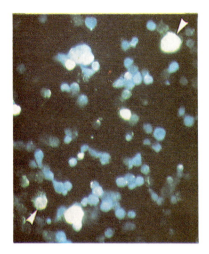 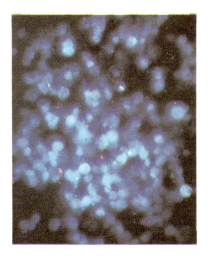

Fig. VII.6. Detection of Epstein-Barr antigens in infected cells by direct immunofluorescence. Infected human fibroblasts were fixed and stained with fluorescein isothiocynate conjugated immunoglobulins in the absence of a counterstain (Fig. VII.1) by the direct method. Arrows showing specific areas of immunofluorescence indicate the presence of cellular antigens. ×2104.

Fig. VII.7. Uninfected control culture incubated for the same time and stained with conjugated immunoglobulins. ×2104.

Chapter 60
Tests for Immunofluorescence

The examination of infected cell cultures by immunofluorescence is the most rapid means of obtaining a viral diagnosis. Infected cells are prepared for examination as described in Chapter 59, but after fixing, the preparation is stained with fluorescein isothiocyanate-conjugated immunoglobulins by either the direct or the indirect method.

The use of the indirect method, involving the use of a preparation of conjugated anti-species immunoglobulins has advantages for the diagnostic laboratory. It is more sensitive than the direct method and avoids the need to maintain a battery of conjugated antisera for the differentiation of all antigenic types of a particular virus group. The application of immunofluorescence

for the Epstein-Barr virus, a herpesvirus, is demonstrated in Fig. VII.6, Fig. VII.7.

Specific areas of immunofluorescence may be highlighted by the use of immunofluorescent counter-stains such as Rhodamine Albumin or Evan's Blue.

Chapter 61
Embryonated Eggs

Certain tissues of the developing chick embryo provide an inexpensive, yet highly effective means of isolating many viruses. The tissues used include (a) the chorion, (b) the allantoic and amniotic sacs and (c) the yolk sac.

These tissues and the various routes used for inoculation are represented diagrammatically in Fig. VII.8.

1 The Chorion

Often mistakenly referred to as the 'chorio-allantoic membrane' or 'CAM', the chorion may be prepared for inoculation by removing a small portion of shell near an avascular region on the flat surface of the egg nearest the embryo and puncturing the shell at the airsac. The chorion is then separated from the outer shell membrane by the application of gentle suction to the airsac. Viruses of the pox- and herpes virus groups grow on the chorion giving rise to the formation of pocks of characteristic size and morphology after 3–4 days at 35–37°C. Pock formation by vaccinia virus is shown in Fig. VII.9 and an uninfected chorion is shown in Fig. VII.10.

2 The Allantoic and Amniotic Sacs

Prior to 1957, it was necessary to passage isolates of influenza first in the amniotic and then the allantoic sacs of 9–11 day chick embryos in order to produce a detectable virus titre. More recent

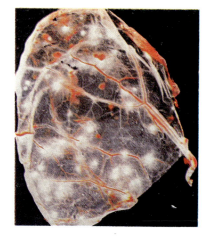

Fig. VII.9. Pock formation by vaccinia virus on the chorion of embryonated eggs. A dilution of vaccinia was inoculated to the prepared chorion of 10 day old chick embryos. After 3 days at 37°C, the chorion was removed and rinsed in saline for examination.

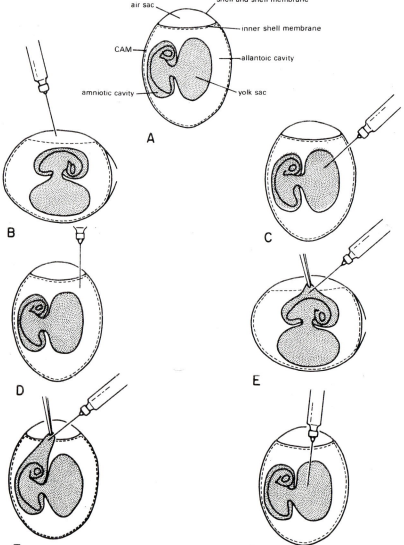

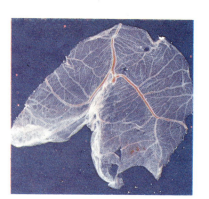

Fig. VII.10. Uninfected chorion incubated for the same time.

Fig. VII.8. Tissues of the developing chick embryo and the various routes of inoculation.

A = Normal egg plus cavities
B = CAM inoculation
C = Yolk sac inoculation
D = Allantoic cavity inoculation
E = Amniotic cavity inoculation
F = Most common route of amniotic cavity inoculation.
G = Most common route of yolk sac inoculation.

influenza isolates do not require preliminary amniotic passage. Allantoic inoculation is still used widely in the diagnosis of influenza but many recent strains have also been shown to grow quite satisfactorily in primate kidney cell cultures, where the presence of virus is detected by haemadsorption.

The growth of influenza viruses in the allantoic cavity is determined after 2 days by removing a small volume of allantoic fluid to a tube or a haemagglutination cup and adding an equal volume of 0.5 per cent chicken red blood cells. The presence of virus is indicated by haemagglutination of these red cells, examples of which are shown in the haemagglutination-inhibition test, see Fig. VII.11, Chapter 64.

3 The Yolk Sac

Although many viruses will grow in the yolk sac of 6–7 day chick embryos, inoculation by this route is seldom used for viral diagnosis. The yolk sac is, however, commonly used for the isolation of rickettsiae.

Chapter 62
Various Other Procedures

1 Animal Hosts

Suckling mice are the only animal hosts used routinely in the diagnosis of viral diseases. Specimens of 0.05 ml are inoculated intracerebrally or intraperitoneally and the animals are examined at daily intervals for symptoms of infection. With certain Coxsackie A viruses, susceptible cell cultures are not available and infection of day old mice results in death due to a generalized myositis within 7 days. For the majority of arthropod-borne viruses (most alpha- and flaviviruses) 1–3 day old mice are the most susceptible hosts and inoculation gives rise to encephalitis, paralysis or death within 7–14 days. Mice inoculated with yellow fever virus exhibit gross

liver necrosis within this period which may be correlated with the formation of specific nuclear inclusion bodies.

2 Immunodiffusion

The differential diagnosis of certain vesicular diseases is possible by tests of immunodiffusion. Vesicular extracts are placed into wells on an agar slide and allowed to react with hyperimmune antisera which is placed in adjacent wells, and a specific reaction is produced by a line of precipitation. The test may be used for the differentiation of varicella and smallpox but relatively large amounts of virus material are required. An immunodiffusion technique is also used for the detection of hepatitis B antigen.

Appropriate positive and negative controls should be run at the same time, see Fig. VII.12 (Chapter 64).

3 Other Tests for the Detection of Hepatitis B Antigen

These include a complement fixation test, an immunoelectrophoresis test, an indirect haemag-glutination test and radioimmunoassay. The latter two tests are more sensitive than the complement fixation and immunodiffusion procedures by factors of several hundred. These tests must now be considered routine for most diagnostic laboratories.

Chapter 63
The Isolation of Viruses of Clinical Significance

A summary of the hosts and isolation procedures most suitable for the diagnosis of infection by differing groups of viruses is presented in Table VII.3.

Table VII.3. Isolation procedures applicable to viruses of clinical significance.

A summary of these procedures is given in the following table:

Virus group and type	No. of serotypes	Host(s) for isolation	Recognition
Picornaviruses:			
Rhinoviruses	>100	HEK, HEF	Picornavirus type CPE at 30–33°C, pH 7.0–7.2. No 1B.
Coxsackie A	24	Day old mice, HEF, PIC (some types)	Extensive myositis within 7 days, CPE
Coxsackie B	6	HEK, HEF, PIC	CPE, IF
Echovirus	31	PIC	CPE, IF
Poliovirus	3	PIC	CPE, IF
Myxoviruses:			
Influenza A	Many	EAM, EAL, PIC	HA, Had
Influenza B	1	EAL	HA
Influenza C	1	EAL	HA
Paramyxoviruses:			
Parainfluenza	4	PIC	IB, Had
Respiratory Syncytial	1	HEp-2 cell lines HEF	CPE, IB, IF
Measles virus	1	PIC, Ham	CPE, IB, Had, IF
Mumps virus	1	HEF, PIC	CPE, IB, Had, IF
Herpesvirus:			
Herpes Simplex	2	HEK	CPE, IB, IF
Varicella/Zoster	1	HEF	CPE, IB, IF
Cytomegalovirus	1	HEF	CPE, IB, IF
Poxviruses:			
Variola (Smallpox)	1	EChor, PIC	Pock morphology CPE, IB, ID
Vaccinia	1	EChor, PIC	Pock morphology CPE, IB, ID
Adenovirus:	33	HEK	CPE, IB
Toga-, Bunya- and Reoviruses:	>200	Suckling mice, Vero and other cell lines	Death, encephalitis, paralysis, CPE, Had, with yellow fever, liver lesions, and IB.
Rhabdovirus:			
Rabies	1	Day old mice	Encephalitis. IF
Hepatitis A:	?1	Marmoset	EM, IEM*
Hepatitis B:	4	Chimpanzee	ID, Serology and Radioimmunoassay.

* EM = electron microscopy.
  IEM = immune EM.

Chapter 64
The Serology of Viral Diseases

In most instances the diagnosis of virus infections is retrospective. Generally, it is not possible to isolate and characterize the infecting agent before the stage of recovery from infection, except where a rapid specific test such as immunofluorescence is employed.

In most cases a positive diagnosis is reached by observing a rise in titre of antibody in sera taken from the patient in the *acute* and *convalescent* stages, usually after a period of 10–14 days.

Four types of serological procedures will be discussed:

1 The Complement Fixation (CF) Test

This test is rapid and inexpensive and provides a means of detecting antibodies common to larger groups of viruses, e.g. to all members of the influenza group. The group-specific antigen is usually an internal component which may be associated with the viral nucleoprotein.

Viral antigens generally consist of clarified cell culture, embryonated egg or mouse brain preparations. With adeno- and poxviruses considerable purification of the antigen can be achieved by treatment of the preparations with fluorocarbons.

The CF test is less sensitive than either the neutralization or haemagglutination inhibition tests. However, because of its broad specificity it is normally one of the first tests used in viral serodiagnosis. CF antibodies are occasionally present at an earlier stage of the infection than other antibodies and also generally decline more rapidly than those detected by other tests.

2 The Neutralization Test

This test is often used after a group identification of the infecting virus has been made by CF test. Mixtures are formed consisting of dilutions of patient's serum and dilutions of a particular virus preparation, calculated to contain approximately two hundred 50 per cent infectious doses (ID_{50}) per 0.1 ml of a stock test virus preparation. Each mixture is allowed to stand for 1–3 hours either at room temperature or at 37°C in order to allow interaction between the virus and any antibody which may be present. After this, 0.1 ml aliquots are then inoculated on to 2–4 susceptible cell cultures in roller-tubes.

The antibody titre for a particular serum is that dilution in a particular mixture which inhibits virus growth in 50 per cent of cell cultures inoculated with aliquots of the mixture. It is calculated from cumulative values obtained over a range of serum dilutions by the Kärber formula. The presence of virus is detected by observing the presence of a CPE haemadsorption or determined by an immunofluorescence test.

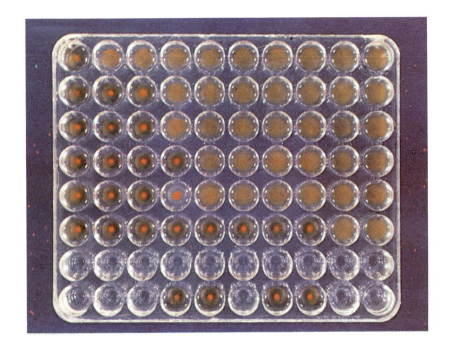

Fig. VII.11. Detection of antibody titres in paired sera by haemagglutination-inhibition tests. The antibody response to influenza vaccination is shown in the paired sera from 3 patients. A sub-unit vaccine was prepared against influenza strain A2/Northern Territory/68 (H3 N2) and haemagglutination-inhibition tests were carried out on sera collected prior to and 3 weeks after vaccination. Inhibitors were removed by treatment with sodium metaperiodate and twofold dilutions prepared in phosphate buffered saline. Four haemagglutinating doses of the same virus were added to each cup and the trays shaken and left for 30 minutes at room temperature. One drop of 5 per cent chicken red blood cells was then added to each cup and the trays reshaken and examined after an additional 35 minutes at room temperature. A small increase in antibody titre representing a primary response can be seen in the paired sera for patient 1, an insignificant response (less than fourfold increase) in patient 2, and a booster or secondary response in patient 3. Negative controls consisting of diluent and red cells above are shown in the lower four cups.

The neutralization test is very sensitive and is used for the final identification of viral sero-types. Neutralizing antibodies are generally produced somewhat later in the infection than CF antibodies and decline more slowly.

3   The Haemagglutination Inhibition (HAI) Test

This test is widely used for the determination of antibody levels against haemagglutinating viruses and has the combined advantages of being rapid, inexpensive and very sensitive.

Dilutions of antibody are prepared in haemagglutination trays and mixed with an equal volume of virus. The latter is normally diluted to contain 4 haemagglutinating doses. After allowing time for virus and antibody (if present) to interact, a drop of a suspension of suitable red blood cells is added to each mixture.

The titre of the serum is the highest dilution which prevents the occurrence of haemagglutination. An example of such a test for influenza is shown in Fig. VII.11.

With most viruses it is necessary first to treat sera with sodium metaperiodate or receptor destroying enzyme (RDE) in order to remove non-specific inhibitors, which would otherwise mask the presence of antibody.

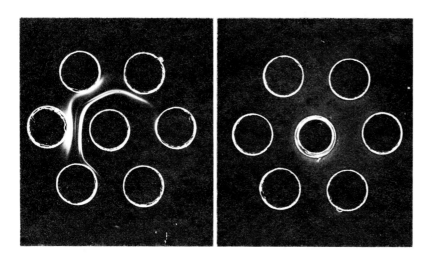

Fig. VII.12. Measurement of antibody titres by immunodiffusion. A pattern of holes was punched in a specially prepared agar slide. An antigen extract was placed in the centre well and twofold dilutions of antisera ranging from 1/2 to 1/16 were placed in surrounding wells. The slide was incubated in a humidified atmosphere at 37°C for 3 days. Specific precipitin lines indicating the presence of several antigens can be seen on the left. A negative control antigen was used on the right.

4   The Immunodiffusion Test

Immunodiffusion tests are less sensitive than the others described above but have the advantages of being rapid and relatively simple to perform requiring only small volumes of sera and test antigens.

A pattern of holes is punched in a thin layer of agar on a specially prepared slide. The test antigen is placed in a central well and dilutions of the test sera in the surrounding wells. The presence of antibody is determined by the occurrence of precipitin lines at the varying dilutions. A typical pattern of precipitin lines for viral antigens is shown on the left side in Fig. VII.12, while no reaction has occurred with the antisera on the right side in Fig. VII.12.

In a modification of the test for the rapid diagnosis of smallpox, hyperimmune serum is placed in the central well and extracts of encrusted vesicles in some of the peripheral wells. A control antigen preparation is also included in one peripheral well and a positive diagnosis is shown by the formation of precipitin lines adjacent to the test and control wells.

Index

T   ook is to b

6·05